Antiviral Drugs - Intervention Strategies

Edited by Farid A. Badria

Published in London, United Kingdom

Antiviral Drugs - Intervention Strategies
http://dx.doi.org/10.5772/intechopen.96839
Edited by Farid A. Badria

Contributors
Farid A. Badria, Mohammad Asif, Saad Alghamdi, Radi Alsafi, Mohammed Othman Aljahdali, Mohammad Habibur Rahman Molla, Foysal Ahammad, Nikhat Farhana, Mohammed Gulzar Ahmed, Mohammed Asif Iqbal, Nishmitha Gretta D'Souza, Sudhina Makuttan, Abdul Rahamanulla, Natasha Naval Aggarwal

First published in London, United Kingdom, 2022 by IntechOpen
IntechOpen is the global imprint of INTECHOPEN LIMITED, registered in England and Wales, registration number: 11086078, 5 Princes Gate Court, London, SW7 2QJ, United Kingdom

British Library Cataloguing-in-Publication Data
A catalogue record for this book is available from the British Library

Additional hard and PDF copies can be obtained from orders@intechopen.com

Antiviral Drugs - Intervention Strategies
Edited by Farid A. Badria
p. cm.
Print ISBN 978-1-80355-330-6
Online ISBN 978-1-80355-331-3
eBook (PDF) ISBN 978-1-80355-332-0

Meet the editor

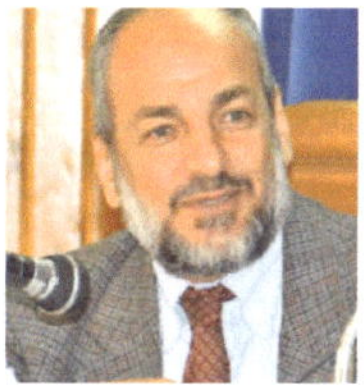

Professor Farid A. Badria was listed among the top 2% of most-cited scientists in medicinal and biomolecular chemistry by Stanford University, USA, in 2019 and 2020. He is the recipient of numerous awards, including The World Academy of Sciences Prize for Public Understanding of Science; the World Intellectual Property Organization Gold Medal (best inventor); State Outstanding Award in Medicine; Outstanding Arab Scholar, Kuwait; and Khawrazmi International Award, Iran. He has also been a scholar of the Arab Development Fund, Kuwait; International Cell Research Organization- United Nations Educational, Scientific and Cultural Organization (ICRO-UNESCO), Chile; and UNESCO Biotechnology France. Professor Badria has more than 250 publications, including 12 books, 20 patents, and several marketed pharmaceutical products to his credit. He continues to lead research projects on developing new therapies for the liver, skin disorders, and cancer.

Contents

Preface

SARS-CoV-2 has several targets that are essential for viral transcription and replication. Therefore, their inhibition could disrupt the virus' life cycle. Among these targets are viral proteases and RNA helicase. SARS-CoV-2 has two proteases, the papain-like protease (PLpro) and the 3-chymotrypsin-like protease (3CLpro), also known as the main protease (Mpro). They are cysteine proteases responsible for the proteolytic processing of the polyproteins that are translated from the viral RNA. PLpro was reported to be responsible for the cleavage of the N-terminus of the viral polyprotein at three cleavage sites, leading to the production of non-structural proteins nsp1-3. Mpro was reported to catalyze the polyprotein cleavage at about eleven sites. This proteolytic process is essential for the production of the functional proteins responsible for viral replication. Moreover, PLpro was reported to be involved in suppressing the host immune response by causing de-ubiquitination and de-ISGylation of the host proteins. Therefore, these enzymes are significant targets for antiviral drugs against coronaviruses and their inhibitors would represent promising antiviral drug candidates.

This book includes five chapters that address several interesting and new approaches regarding non-conventional intervention strategies for viral infection, particularly SARS-CoV-2.

Chapter 1 is an introductory chapter on intervention therapeutic strategies against SARS-CoV-2. Chapter 2 discusses the repurposing of natural products to target COVID-19, including molecular targets and new avenues for drug discovery. Chapter 3 examines antiviral drugs and their roles in the treatment of coronavirus infection. Chapter 4 presents immunoinformatics and computer-aided drug design as novel approaches against emerging and re-emerging infectious diseases. Finally, Chapter 5 discusses the repurposing, repositioning, and reprofiling of antiviral agents to combat viral infections.

This book poses a balance between developments in scientific research and the premise that researchers must be able to absorb and link scientific advances with clinical practice so that the management of diseases can be based on sound physiological concepts.

Farid A. Badria, Ph.D.
Liver Research Lab, FAB-Lab,
Faculty of Pharmacy,
Pharmacognosy Department,
Mansoura University,
Mansoura, Egypt

Chapter 1

Introductory Chapter: An Intervention Therapeutic Strategies against SARS-CoV-2

Farid A. Badria

1. Introduction

The objectives of this introductory chapter is to outline the possible intervention therapeutic strategies against SARS-CoV-2.

Upon such vision, all research projects, scientific creations, trouble-shooting and problem-solving techniques must be based on healthy environment. As a matter of fact, the environment has provided us with the best of everything, of food, water, air, and a cure for every illness. In our turn, we should make good use of God's blessings bestowed upon us through natural sources by which we can fight contagious diseases including COVID-19.

Accordingly, the founding factors of this vision will be:

- Protect the environment against all hazards.
- Treat the current diseases by introducing totally indigenous thought, ideas, raw materials and technology to produce a safe, effective, and economic therapy.
- Spread hygienic awareness and good sound health practices as a protection against potential dangers.

The premises of this vision are:

- ○ A sound healthy environment embraces a sound and healthy society.
- ○ A healthy environment provides us with a cure to any ailment.
- ○ An unhealthy environment is the source of all illnesses.

2. A possible approach for intervention of SARS-CoV-2 infectivity

SARS-CoV-2 genomic RNA is protected by two envelopes: phospholipid bilayer and protein. The human cell entry by the virus was prompted upon S-protein (Spike protein), which resides in the envelope anchors to ACE2. Protease cleaved the S-protein into S-1 and S-2 fragments, whereas S-1 binds to ACE2. While S-2 was cleaved by serine protease enzyme (TMPRSS2), leading to membrane fusion. This may halt the first step of infection with the virus, as presented in **Figure 1**.

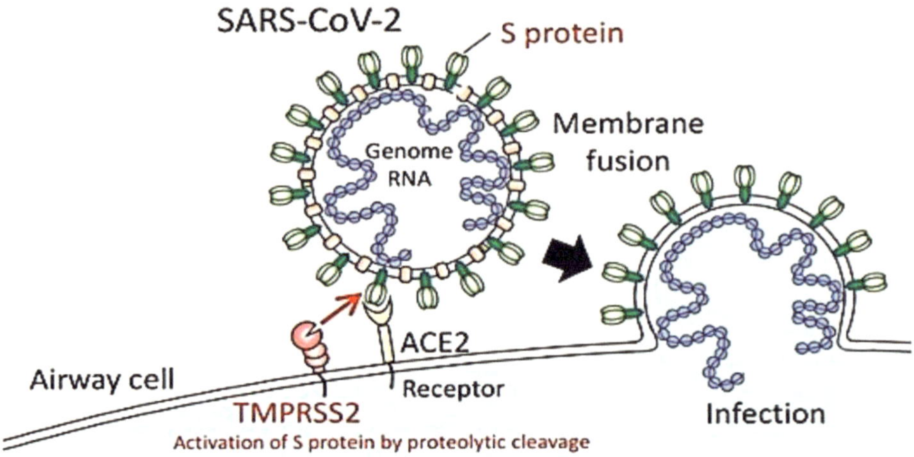

Figure 1.
SARS-CoV-2 entry to the host cell (airway cell) that initiates with the S-protein on its envelope and the endocytosis process. This illustrates the essentiality of ACE2 and TMPRSS2 in the SARS-CoV-2 infection.

3. Promising natural serine protease inhibitors

Serine proteases, including elastase, trypsin, and chymotrypsin, are a large class of enzymes and play various roles in human health, including blood coagulation and immune response. An increase or decrease in protease activity can induce pathologies, including inflammation, cancer, stroke, heart attack, and pancreatitis.

3.1 Halting of viral replication

3.1.1 Inhibition of SARS-CoV-2 NSP15 endoribonuclease

Nidoviral RNA uridylate-specific endoribonuclease (NendoU) is one of the enigmatic enzymes that is corresponding to Nsp15, carrying a C-terminal catalytic domain (EndoU family). They perform various biological functions related to RNA processing. All characterized family members display an RNA endonuclease activity [1].

Inhaled ciclesonide is expected to reduce viral replication and host inflammation in the lungs, with decreased immunosuppressive effects compared to systemic corticosteroids, as ciclesonide primarily remains in the lung tissue, and does not significantly enter the bloodstream. This is also considered to be another example of drug repurposing. Therefore, we could conclude that natural steroids are potential inhibitors [2].

3.1.2 SARS-CoV-2 main protease inhibitors (M^{pro} = $3CL^{pro}$)

There are many examples of α-keto amides inhibitors of natural origin, such as eurystatin A and B (prolyl endopeptidase inhibitor), complestatin (HIV replication inhibitor), and aplidine (antitumor) (**Figure 2**) [3].

4. The immunomodulation effect

The immunomodulation effect may be useful in controlling the cytokine storm that occurs late among critically ill SARS-CoV-2 infected patients.

It was reported among several patients. A noticeable elevation of both IL-6 and IL-10 levels in response to SARS-CoV-2 infection. Virus results in the increase in cytokines IL-6 and IL-10 [4]. This immune reaction may lead to a cytokine storm then followed by a failure of several body organs, which may lead to death. It was suggested that some chloroquine derivatives may retain immunomodulatory activity and may be able to subdue the reactions of an immune response. This may help in early intervention as well as avoid the most likely bad scenario of the infection to a life-threatening status [5].

Pro-inflammatory cytokines, for example, IL-6 and IL-10, may result in expression induced by LPS. However, modulating several intracellular signaling pathways in macrophages and halting LPS-induced cytokines production by decreasing the mRNA stability by suppressing ERK1/2 activation. This hypothesis could be accomplished by a series of naturally isolated compounds, for example, luteolin, syringic acid, apigenin, curcumin, and lichochalcone, at the transcriptional level [6].

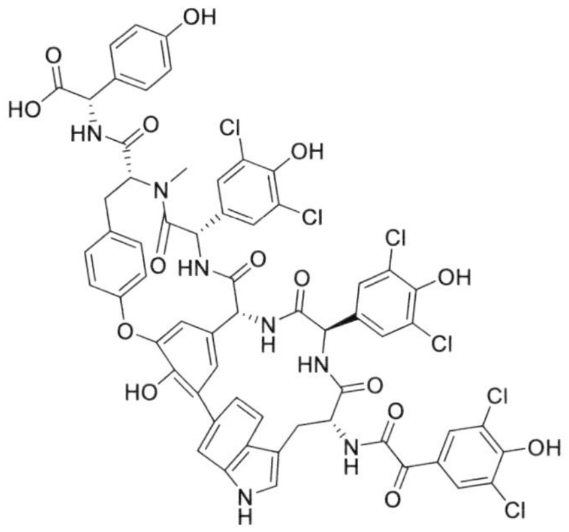

Complestatin

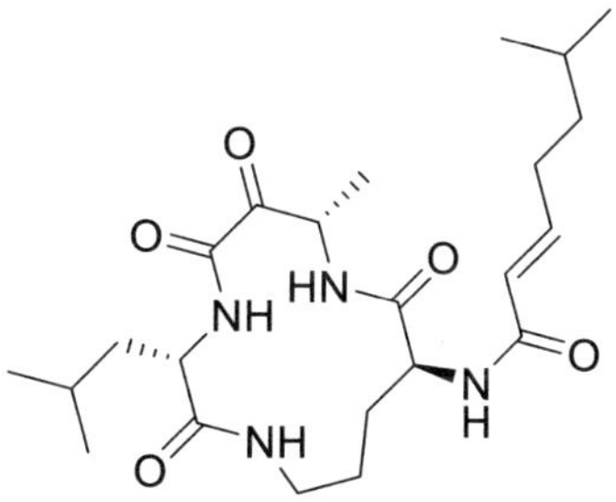

Eurystatin A

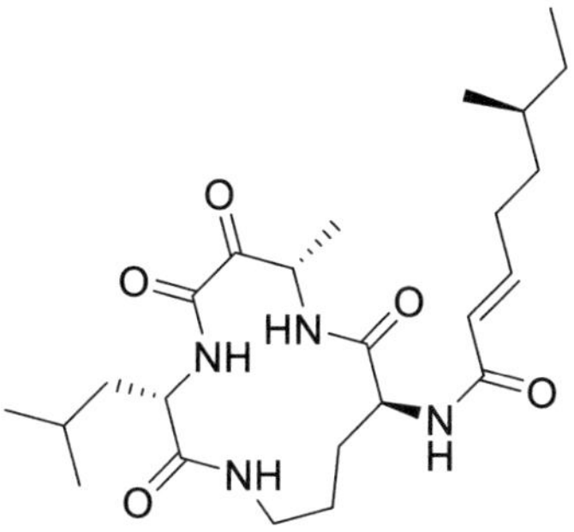

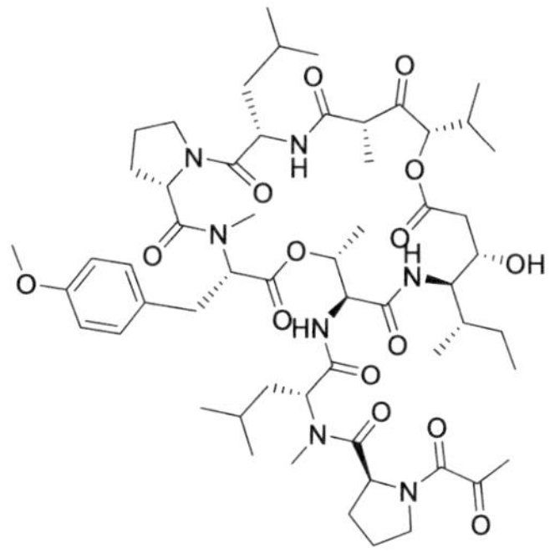

Figure 2.
Natural alpha-ketoamides could be used as strong inhibitors of viral proteases (M^{pro}).

In *conclusion*, there is always hope to find potent, safe, and economic therapeutic agents for the treatment and management of COVID-19 outbreak from the commonly abundant natural products, such as phytosterols, alpha-ketoamides, and flavonoids. However, these findings need further investigation and experimental studies to be approved, but this could open the door for the utilization of abundantly available natural products to provide a therapeutic strategy via developing safe, effective, and economic drugs against this pandemic.

Author details

Farid A. Badria
Faculty of Pharmacy, Pharmacognosy Department, Mansoura University, Liver Research Lab (FAB-Lab), Mansoura, Egypt

*Address all correspondence to: faridbadria@gmail.com; badri002@mans.edu.eg

References

[1] Ulferts R, Ziebuhr J. Nidovirus ribonucleases: Structures and functions in viral replication. RNA Biology. 2011;**8**:295-304

[2] Matsuyama S, Kawase M, Nao N, Shirato K, Ujike M, Kamitani W, et al. The inhaled corticosteroid ciclesonide blocks coronavirus RNA replication by targeting viral NSP15. bioRxiv. 2020 Dec 9;**95**(1):e01648-e01720

[3] Muthukumar A, Sangeetha S, Sekar G. Recent developments in functionalization of acyclic α-keto amides. Organic & Biomolecular Chemistry. 2018;**16**: 7068-7083

[4] Huang C, Wang Y, Li X, Ren L, Zhao J, Hu Y, et al. Clinical features of patients infected with 2019 novel coronavirus in Wuhan, China. The Lancet. 2020;**395**: 497-506

[5] Yao X, Ye F, Zhang M, Cui C, Huang B, Niu P, et al. In vitro antiviral activity and projection of optimized dosing design of hydroxychloroquine for the treatment of severe acute respiratory syndrome coronavirus 2 (SARS-CoV-2). Clinical Infectious Diseases. 2020 Jul 28;**71**(15):732-739

[6] Grigore A. Plant phenolic compounds as immunomodulatory agents. In: Phenolic Compounds–Biological Activity. London, UK: IntechOpen; 2017. pp. 75-98

Chapter 2

Perspective Chapter: Repurposing Natural Products to Target COVID-19 – Molecular Targets and New Avenues for Drug Discovery

Farid A. Badria

Abstract

World Health Organization (WHO) declared on March 11, 2020, coronavirus disease, which erupted in December 19th, 2019 in Wuhan, China (COVID-19) as worldwide pandemic disease. Researchers worldwide were successful to provide a prophylactic approach *via* developing several vaccines, which were swiftly approved by WHO under Emergency Use Listing (EUL) status. So far, lopinavir, chloroquine, azithromycin, hydroxychloroquine, favipiravir, umifenovir, ribavirin, remdesivir, and darunavir have been tested clinically. Hydroxychloroquine, favipiravir, and chloroquine exhibited a high ratio of distribution for the lung and were reported to minimize viral tonnage in respiratory system of many COVID-19 cases. However, none of the tested drugs showed a conclusive, safe, and efficient activity against COVID-19. This prompted many experts in drug discovery to fetch in the treasure of many available old drugs of natural origin to repurpose based upon their well-studied pharmacology, pharmacodynamics, virtual screening, and artificial intelligence studies. In this review chapter, we will address the repurposing of natural products and their derivatives to be used in treatment of COVID-19 *via* targeting host cells machinery and viral proteins either in early stages by blocking virus entry to cells or lately through inhibition of viral replication.

Keywords: COVID-19, inflammation, viral replication, drug repurposing, artificial intelligence, natural products

1. Introduction

SARS-CoV-2 is a relatively large virus with single-stranded RNA genome, belongs to beta coronaviruses that affects the lower respiratory system to cause viral pneumonia. The gastrointestinal system, kidney, heart, liver, and central nervous system may also be attacked leading to multiple organ failure. It is surrounded by an envelope composed of a lipid bilayer and envelope proteins [1].

1.1 The life cycle of COVID-19

The COVID-19 viral infection is mediated by three main stages: the first one involves host cell entry through endocytosis and transportation proteins; the second stage initiates viral RNA translation to polyprotein, which is subjected to cleavage by the main viral proteinases Mpro and Papain-like proteases PLpro to produce the effector proteins; in the final stage, the negative-strand viral RNA is translocated to the Golgi apparatus to produce new virions, and the newly produced virus are released by exocytosis [1].

1.2 Host cell viral entry and nuclear translocation

The viral entry was found to be mediated by endocytic pathways, which is initiated by the binding of spike protein (S protein), a protein found on the envelope of the virus, to a receptor protein located on the host cell surface membrane, known as angiotensin-converting enzyme 2 (ACE2). The S protein is cleaved into S1 and S2 by a human cell-derived protease that is assumed to be Furin. S1 then binds to its receptor, ACE2. The other fragment, S2, is cleaved by TMPRSS2, a serine protease. Thus, ACE2 and TMPRSS2 are essential in airway cells for SARS-CoV-2 infection [2].

Also the viral entry was found to be facilitated through endocytosis [3], especially clathrin-mediated endocytosis (CME) helps in translocation of ACE-2/virus complex to endosome where the virus is uncoated by the action of acidic proteases such as cathepsins, which are cysteine proteases in host cells involved in facilitating viral entry of several viruses such as SARS-COV and MERS-COV [4]. It's worthy to note that cathepsins are also involved in S protein cleavage [5, 6].

After uncoating, the viral RNA expression and replication require subcellular localization of viral and cellular proteins from cytoplasm to the nucleus. The viral infection induces the translocation and expression of group of suprafamily protein in the host cells called karyopherin, Importins (IMP) α/β heterodimer. These proteins are reported to be utilized by the virus not only for translocation purposes, but also for disruption of self-antiviral defenses in response to interferon via intervening with the nuclear import of signal transducer and activator of transcription proteins (STAT). Chromosome Region Maintenance-1 (CRM1) is one of those proteins that contribute significantly in nuclear export of viral protein and RNA in wide range of viruses [7].

1.3 Translation of viral RNA to nonstructural protein

The SARS-Cov-2 genome has a large replicase gene, which contains nonstructural proteins (NSPs), structural proteins, and accessory genes. The replicase gene encodes two open reading frames (ORFs) after frameshifting, translated into two large polyproteins pp1a and pp1ab, then processed by two viral proteases: papain-like protease (PLpro, encoded within Nsp3) and Mpro aslo called 3C-like protease (3CLpro, encoded by Nsp5) to produce 16 viral Nsps that their function has been linked to RNA replication. PLpro is believed to play important role to protect the virus from immune response by inactivating ubiquitin-dependent cellular responses to viral infection and blocking of cytokine production [8, 9].

1.4 Genome replication and production of new viruses

After cell invasion, a full-length negative-strand RNA template is synthesized by nonstructural protein 12 (Nsp12) RNA-dependent RNA polymerase (RdRp) to produce more viral genomic RNA [10].

Another important nonstructural protein is RNA helicase, which has main role in the replication of viruses by catalyze unwinding of double-stranded RNA. It is structurally conserved among different types of viruses, thereby making it an excellent target for development of broad-spectrum antiviral agents [11, 12].

1.5 Translation of structural protein virion assembly and release

In this stage, the viral RNA is translocated to endoplasmic reticulum (ER) where it is translated to transmembrane structural proteins (S, HE, M, and E) and some membrane-associated accessory proteins, except for the N protein, which is translated by free ribosomes in the cytoplasm [13]. These structural proteins play the main role in virion morphogenesis and the structural components recruitment to the proper assembly site. Then they are released from the cell by exocytosis by the help of several host factors [14].

However, in the COVID-19 pandemic, an integrated approach encompassing prophylaxis, diagnosis, and treatment must be adopted worldwide.

2. Approaches for prophylaxis, diagnosis, and therapy

Among the top priorities for regulating and monitoring COVID-19 are:

1. An appropriate prophylactic procedure (vaccination).

2. Accurate diagnostic battery.

3. An unambiguous therapeutic regimen.

2.1 An appropriate prophylactic procedure (vaccination)

WHO stated that "vaccine must supply a quite convenient beneficial environment for dealing with jeopardy; with high performance, only passing with mild effects and with no danger effects." The vaccine should be appropriate for lactating, gravid women and for all ages and has many production sources dwell in high-, middle-, and low-income countries [15]. There is a race among several pharmaceutical companies to provide a treatment for COVID-19. Unfortunately, this completion had led to a big controversy, which was refuted by WHO issued on 20 November 2020 "there is a conditional recommendation against the use of remdesivir since there isn't enough evidence to support its use." Moreover, WHO has issued a conditional recommendation against the use of remdesivir in hospitalized patients, regardless of disease severity, as there is currently no evidence that remdesivir improves survival and other outcomes in these patients (https://www.who.int/news-room/feature-stories/detail/who-recommends-against-the-use-of-remdesivir-in-covid-19-patients).

However, by the end of 2020 (exactly December 2020), Pfizer/BioNTech was able to get an Emergency Use Listing approval (EUL) for vaccine against COVID-19. Currently and as reported by on January 20th, 2022, nine vaccines were granted EUL status [16, 17].

- The Pfizer/BioNTech Comirnaty vaccine, 31 December 2020.

- The SII/COVISHIELD and AstraZeneca/AZD1222 vaccines, 16 February 2021.
- The Janssen/Ad26.COV 2.S vaccine developed by Johnson & Johnson, 12 March 2021.
- The Moderna COVID-19 vaccine (mRNA 1273), 30 April 2021.
- The Sinopharm COVID-19 vaccine, 7 May 2021.
- The Sinovac-CoronaVac vaccine, 1 June 2021.
- The Bharat Biotech BBV152 COVAXIN vaccine, 3 November 2021.
- The Covovax (NVX-CoV2373) vaccine, 17 December 2021.
- The Nuvaxovid (NVX-CoV2373) vaccine, 20 December 2021

2.2 Diagnosis

2.2.1 Clinical laboratory

- The clinical laboratory is an important and essential tool for the diagnosis, follow-up, and evolution, as well as in the prognosis of any pathology that is active or not. In the COVID-19 pandemic, several biomarkers' involvement as indicators of the disease's current state has been reported, while others have proved to be useful prognostic markers. Some of these characteristics are as follows [18].
- General laboratory findings in SARS-CoV-2 infection sometimes indicate leukocytosis or leukopenia, with marked lymphopenia in the disease's first stages. Besides, the neutrophilia presence has been related to an unfavorable prognosis [19].
- Thrombocytopenia, lymphopenia, thrombocytopenia, D-dimer, elevated C-reactive protein (CRP) (happened repeatedly in critical cases), and leukopenia are not distinctive laboratory factors [20].
- COVID-19 patients who have diabetes mellitus of type 2 (T2DM) expressed minimized levels of lymphocytes, body mass index (BMI), albumin, and uric acid (UA), and increased CRP levels. The reduced levels of albumin, UA, and BMI may be related to nutritional consumption and oxidative stress response. The increased CRP levels and decreased lymphocyte counts may be related to the infection [21].

2.2.2 Imaging

Medical imaging, such as Computed Tomography (CT) and X-ray, plays a significant function in the combat against the pandemic. So, the current AI methods can be used to help medical specialists and strengthen imaging tools. Also, AI could also increase work performance by effective detection of CT and X-ray diseases. The Computer-Aided Diagnosis (CAD) models enable physicians to take correct clinical choices on disease diagnosis, monitoring, and prognosis [22]. Many radiological characteristics are used to categorize the disease and help in discovering the treatment, such as the following:

- The most direct method to identify the degree of disease is imaging, as it is effective and accurate. Consolidation and diffuse lesions are features of severe pneumonia. Doubled ground-glass opacity, unification, and interlobular septal thick ply in the right and left lungs are the popular chest CT discoveries for COVID-19, which are particularly spread under the pleura. The serious part of the pandemic diagnosis and examination is computed tomography [23].

- A sensitive examination method is called spiral CT. It can be used for diagnosis in the early stages and estimation of development. This method has diagnostic allergy and precision preferable to the disclosure of nucleic acid [24]. During the first week of the illness, appearance and blended predominance with opacity in the lower lung are quite dubious of COVID-19. However, few illness cases may have a normal chest outcome despite positive testing for COVID-19 [25].

- The proportion of infected cases with mild COVID-19 symptoms was relatively high-rise. Misdiagnosis in some cases can result from checking for COVID-19 with only chest CT, which would result in a possibility of contagion risk. It was not appropriate as a separate screening device. Visual, quantitative interpretation depended on CT images with great diagnostic capability and good matchmaking. It can help in clinical classification; it is predictable to strictly evaluate the severe COVID-19 cases and combining with the clinical information to guide the clinical treatment [26].

2.3 Therapy

Therapeutic interferences can be categorized into four main classes: general treatment, antiviral treatments, particular medications, and other medications.

The effectiveness and safety of COVID-19 have been tested using several drugs, such as chloroquine, remdesivir, favipiravir, and hydroxychloroquine. Some of them had presented antiviral impacts against COVID-19 but no conclusive evidences [27].

Although the serious disease has been related to hyperinflammation induced by COVID-19, the immune responses of acute COVID-19 stay ambiguous. Some researchers comprehensively analyzed circumferential immune troubles in blood for 42 recovered and infected by COVID-19. The activation of various immune strains is recognized, including oligoclonal plasmablast expansion, trafficking receptor modulation on granulocytes, innate lymphocytes, and T cell activation, which separated acute COVID-19 patients or moderate-severe patients from healthy donors or COVID-19-recovered. One of the predictive biomarkers is the ratio between neutrophil and lymphocyte of organ failure and disease gravity. Results appeared wide innate and adaptive leukocyte annoyances that characterize dysregulated have an infection in extreme COVID-19 disease, and medication examination is required. There were no efficacious antiviral medications, even common drugs with strong effect as abidol, ritonavir/lopinavir showed no exceptional impact on clinical progression, virus clearance, or deaths [28].

The meta-analysis of corticosteroid treatment and available observational studies suggested maximized death rates and subaltern contagion rates in influenza, maximized viremia, weakened antibody response, and weakened infection riddance MERS-CoV and SARS-CoV, and corticosteroid treatment complications in recovered patients [29]. Therefore, in the medication of COVID-19, corticosteroids should not be supported or even applied for acute patients.

The plasma of convalescent for severe influenza infection and SARS-CoV medication was proposed to minimize the mortality rate and days number in hospital, particularly after symptom appearance and administered plasma early [30].

As for inoculation, if any cross-reactive epitopes were recognized among COVID-19 and SARS-CoV, the preceding vaccine of SARS-CoV might be reused to expedite the COVID-19 vaccine progression. It is recommended for prophylaxis, streptococcus pneumonia, and influenza vaccination, especially in the elderly [31].

2.4 Drug repurposing and COVID-19

Drug repurposing is also a quick tool that creates a shortcut to find a safe and effective therapy for this exciting pandemic. It depends on the fact that their safety profile, side effects, posology, and drug interactions are well known [27]. Currently, several FDA-approved drugs are tested for their potential to treat COVID-19 infection such as lopinavir, chloroquine, azithromycin, hydroxychloroquine, favipiravir, umifenovir, ribavirin, remdesivir, and darunavir have been tested in many COVID-19 clinical experiments for hopeful use under emergency protocol. Unfortunately, none of these tested drugs showed a conclusive results and satisfactory outcomes among treated patients. Therefore, several studies used in silico tools for prediction of the ability of drugs to interact with molecular targets important for viral replications.

In that aspect, the liver research laboratory (FAB-Lab, Faculty of Pharmacy, Mansoura University, Mansoura, Egypt) has applied several approaches for not only improving the pharmacological effect of easily accessible natural products, but also identifying new applications for them. Drug repositioning or repurposing may reveal a new approach to rediscover new uses for clinically approved existing old drugs [32]. This book revealed the theory, applications, and/or hazardous outcomes on drug discovery in different disciplines in medicine; e.g. dermatology [33, 34], cancer [35–37], and neurological disorders [38].

A hopeful mechanism to cure COVID-19 patients is the reusing of trusted antiviral treatments in opposition to COVID-19. Viral loads are reduced by employing the antiviral treatments that have risen lung allocations, which is helpful to COVID-19 cases. There are a number of antiviral medications such as [39].

2.4.1 Natural products inhibitors for targeting COVID-19

Some results depended on molecular docking and network direct pharmacology action on COVID-19, for examples:

- Kaempferol, aloe-emodin, quercetin, luteolin, forsythoside E, rutin, and hyperoside in Lianhua Qinwen might be the buoyant components in hindering COVID-19 by computer-assisted treatment design (CADD) of virtual checking and network pharmacology analysis through JAK-STAT signaling pathway [40–42].

- Patchouli alcohol, saikosaponin ergosterol, 23-acetate alisol B, shionone, B (Bupleuri Radix) could act straight on the COVID-19 3CL pro to restrain infection multiplication. On differentiate, shionone (Asteris Radix et Rhizoma), tussilagone, patchouli alcohol, asarinin, ephedrine hydrochloride, and ergosterol might work on steward cells ACE2 to restrain the attack [43–46].

- Licorice glycoside E, (2R)-7-hydroxy-2-(4-hydroxyphenyl) chroman-4-ketone, robinin, naringenin, quercetin, kaempferol, irisolidone, and isorhamnetin from Huoxiang Zhengqi as 3CL pro restraints, which may block COVID-19 repetition by focusing on E2F1 and PIK3CG by PI3K-Akt signaling path [44]. Rosmarinic acid could block virus repetition through the PI3K-Akt signal path [47].

- Quercetin, Kaempferol, luteolin, baicalein, glyasperin C, licochalcone B, and oroxylin A were suggested to tie with organizing different signals paths and ACE2, as BCL2, PTGS2, Kaposi sarcoma-related herpesvirus contagion, CASP3, hepatitis C, Epstein-Barr virus infection, measles, and human cytomegalovirus contagion.

- Baicalein, kaempferol, luteolin, rhubarb wogonin, and quercetin had a great partiality with COVID-19 3CL hydrolase [48].

As previously explained, nonstructural proteins of COVID-19 and several factors and receptors in host cells are essential for viral entry and replication, which means that both should be considered in the process of the development of effective antiviral agents as depicted in **Figure 1**. In this section, we will address known natural products inhibitors to the key targets controlling viral entry and replication.

2.4.1.1 Inhibition of viral invasion process

2.4.1.1.1 Inhibition of SARS-CoV-2 lipid-dependent attachment to host cells

Targeting host lipids is an intriguing antiviral strategy. Coronaviruses are a class of viruses with a lipid envelope that requires a plasma membrane fusion process mediated by endocytosis, a mechanism that involves certain cholesterol-rich micro-domains and its ACE2 receptor [49] and mediates the early stages of internalization of coronaviruses [50].

Macromolecules such as methyl-β-cyclodextrin have been used to inhibit attachment of coronaviruses to host cells. These nontoxic macromolecules mimic attack sites for the enveloped virus, competing with host cell attack sites. It could also decrease ACE2 expression in the cell membrane, thereby reducing the infectivity of coronaviruses, such as SARS-CoV-2 [51].

Natural compounds including phytosterols and triterpenes (**Figure 2**) can exert the same action. For example, betulinic acid also has the same lipophilic properties as cholesterol, so it may therefore compete with cholesterol, replacing it in plasma membranes, or it may bind to the virus instead of raft cholesterol, acting as a soluble competitor [52].

2.4.1.1.2 Blocking the viral entry process by inhibiting TMPRSS2 activity

TMPRSS2, a human cell surface serine protease, results in membrane fusion. ACE2 and TMPRSS2 are essential in airway cells for SARS-CoV-2 infection [53].

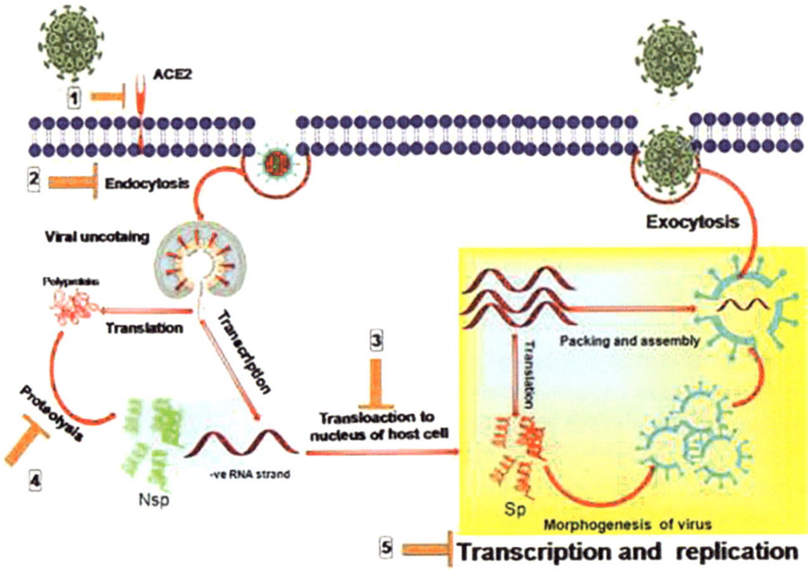

Figure 1.
Different approaches for targeting viral entry and replication of the COVID-19. (1) Inhibition of S protein binding to ACE2, (2) disruption of endocytic pathways, (3) inhibition of nuclear translocation of viral RNA and protein by host cell mediators, (4) inhibition of the proteolysis of viral polyprotein to the nonstructural proteins (Nsp), (5) inhibition of transcription and replication of viral RNA.

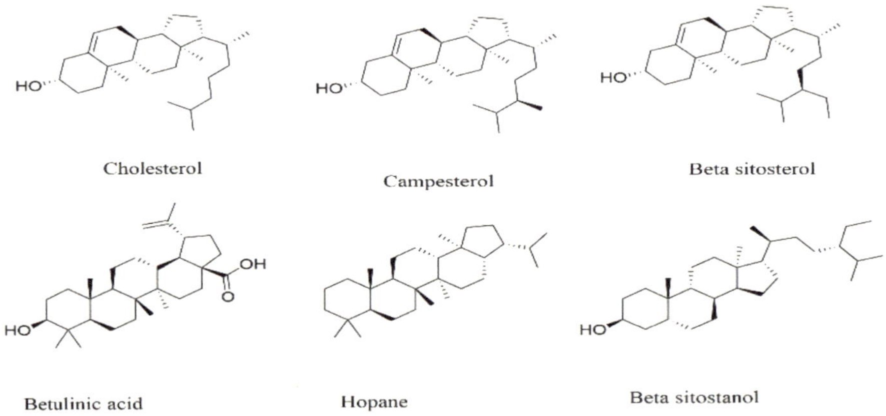

Figure 2.
Chemical structures of the most common phytosterols. They are considered as potential inhibitors of SARS-CoV-2 lipid-dependent attachment to host cells, a possible approach for decreasing its infectivity.

ACE2 inhibition should not be tracked as a treatment strategy as ACE inhibitors upregulate the expression of ACE receptors providing more binding sites for SARS-CoV-2. On the other hand, blocking TMPRSS2 is accessible and will prevent the fusion of the envelope of the virus with host cell surface membranes. Nafamostat, an existing safe drug used for pancreatitis, may inhibit SARS-CoV-2 entry by inhibiting TMPRSS2 activity.

In this context, several reported serine protease inhibitors from nature could be repurposed to target TMPRSS2.

Potent serine protease inhibitors have been reported from filamentous marine cyanobacteria. Most of these molecules are 3-amino-6 hydroxy-piperidone (AHP-containing cyclic depsipeptides). The AHP moiety is crucial for serine protease inhibitory activity, and any structural or conformational variations to this unit will affect activity (**Figure 3**) [54].

2.4.1.1.3 Inhibition of endocytic pathway.

2.4.1.1.3.1 Increase of the endosomal and lysosomal pH using lysosomotropism agents

It's now well established that endocytosis is the nick bottle for COVID-19 entry to the host cells, thus inhibiting this pathway could reduce the infectivity of the virus dramatically. This could be achieved by increasing of the endosomal and lysosomal pH using lysosomotropism agents, which disrupt the proteolytic action of host cell proteases, which work optimally in acidic pH and prevent the cleavage of the S Protein of the virus [55]. While chloroquine (CQ) and its derivative are developed originally for treatment of malaria, but since they demonstrated potent activity by direct acting on the virus and by preventing its endocytosis, they were repurposed for treatment of several viral infection and currently used widely used in therapeutic protocol for treatment of COVID-19 [56]. Bafilomycin A1, a vacuolar-type H^{+-}ATPase inhibitor, lies in the same category and could explain the use of azithromycin, a structurally related macrolide antibiotic for treatment of COVID-19 patients [57].

2.4.1.1.3.2 Cathepsins inhibitors

Inhibition of cysteine proteases such as cathepsins could be an important approach due to their role in viral entry, and luckily the incorporation of these protein in the pathogenesis of several diseases such as cancer, metabolic conditions, and Alzheimer's has led to the discovery and development of several inhibitors that could be repurposed for treatment of COVID-19 infection. E-64, a compound isolated from the fungus *Aspergillus japonicus*, can bind irreversibly to this target without showing

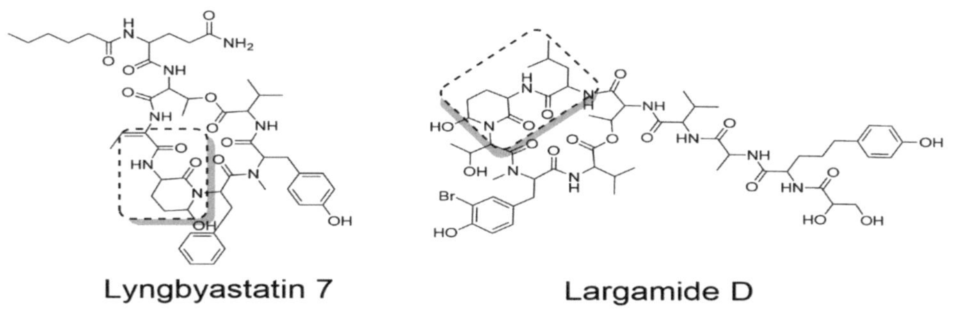

Figure 3.
Serine protease inhibitors isolated from marine cyanobacteria. Potential blockers for the requisite viral entry process (inhibition of the S protein-initiated membrane fusion by inhibiting TMPRSS2 activity).

toxic activity; also gallinamide A and Miraziridine A marine natural products were reported to possess the same activity. There are a number of natural compounds that possess a promising cathepsins inhibition with IC_{50} range from 2 to 10 micromolar, such as panduratin A, guttiferone A, ursolic acid, and agathisflavone [58].

2.4.1.1.3.3 Clathrin-mediated endocytosis (CME) pathway blockage

As addressed earlier, CME is one of the main mechanisms for viral entry; hence, its inhibition could be a reliable method for control of the infection. Ouabain and bufalin cardiotonic steroids, which are used for treatment of cardiovascular diseases, have demonstrated antiviral activity against MERS-CoV infection at nanomolar concentrations by affecting the CME pathway [59]. This is consistent with recent report by Jeon et al., where ouabain, lanatoside C, and digitoxin were able to reduce viral viability of COVID-19 in micromolar concentrations [60].

Bolinaquinone, a sesquiterpenoid derivative with quinone ring, isolated from marine *Dysidea* sp., which is known to possess anti-inflammatory activity, however, affinity chromatography coupled with mass spectrometry revealed the ability of this molecule to inhibit clathrin in a concentration comparable to chlorpromazine, a well-known inhibitor of this target [61]. Also, ikarugamycin, an antibiotic that was found to specifically inhibit CEM effectively [62].

2.4.1.1.4 Inhibition of translocation mechanisms

Like other viruses, COVID-19 uses the replication machinery of the host cell for transcription and replication of Viral RNA; this means that viral materials such as nonstructural proteins and negative-strand RNA should be relocated to the nucleus and endoplasmic reticulum.

2.4.1.1.4.1 Importin (IMP) $\alpha/\beta1$ heterodimer inhibition

Interestingly, ivermectin, an antiparasitic FDA-approved drug, has been reported to inhibit nuclear transport in host cells such as (IMP) $\alpha/\beta1$ heterodimer preventing the translocation of viral DNA integrase in HIV-1 and other viruses. Recently, ivermectin has shown potent antiviral activity against COVID-19 [63]. In fact, such effect was linked to the broad-spectrum antiviral activity of this molecule [64].

2.4.1.1.4.2 Chromosomal maintenance 1 (CRM-1 also known as exportin 1 (XPO1)) inhibition

Finally, leptomycin B (LMB), a compound isolated from *Streptomyces* sp, with prominent anticancer and anti-inflammatory activity, which is attributed to its ability to block CRM-1. While the main research focus of this target was on its role in tumorigenesis; it's now known that it contributes in the infection of different viruses. There are a lot of natural compounds reported to target CRM-1 such as valtrate, which is anxiolytic compound isolated from valerian roots, acetoxychavicol, curcumin, goniothalamin, piperlongumine, and plumbagin. These compounds share the presence of alpha, beta unsaturated ketone, making structure similarly to LMB, which seems to be important feature to interact with Cys528 via Michael-type addition and exert their inhibitory actions. Despite the reported antiviral activity of these molecules, there are

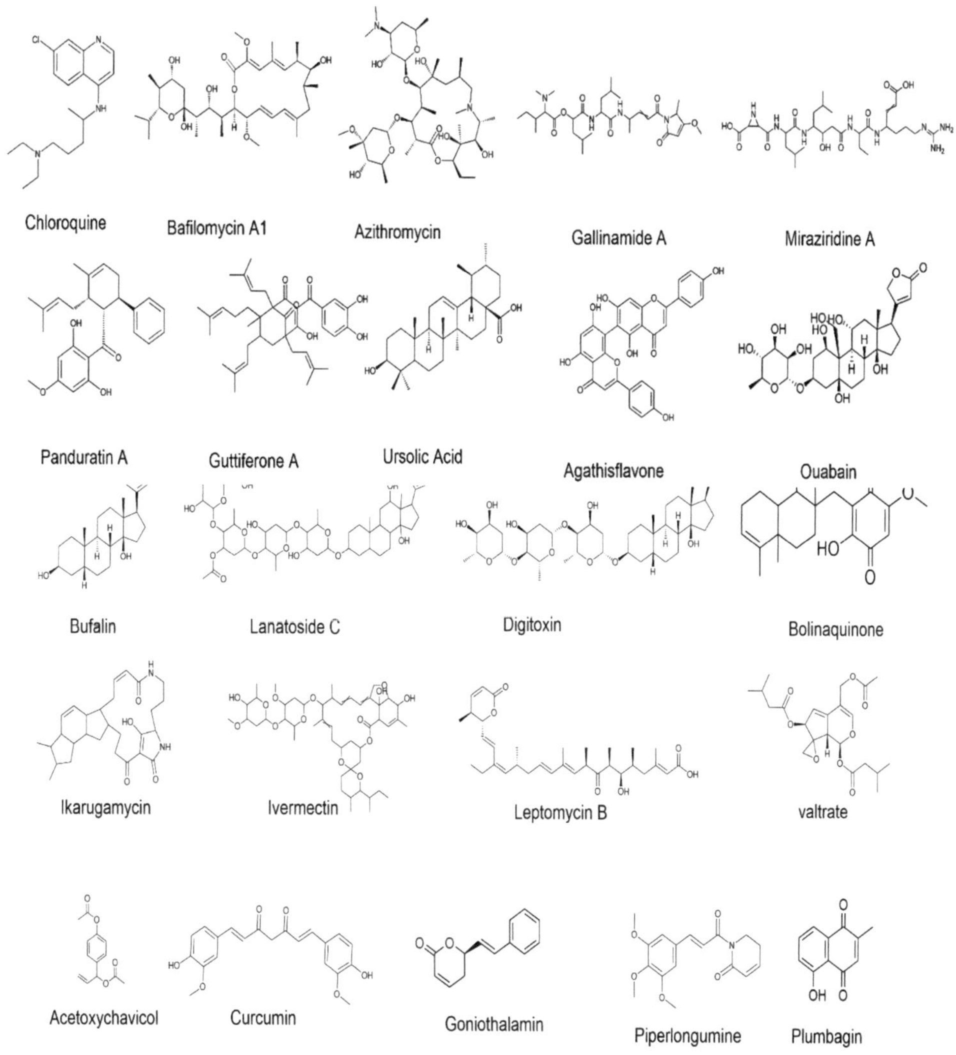

Figure 4.
Chemical structure of compounds that inhibit endocytic pathway and translocation mechanisms.

no studies addressing this effect in COVID-19. **Figure 4** shows the chemical structure of compounds that inhibit endocytic pathway and translocation mechanisms.

2.4.1.2 Inhibition of nonstructural proteins formation

We have addressed the role of host cells factor and protein inhibition in controlling viral infection. So, we will focus mainly on some important targets of the virus itself. The proteolysis of polypeptide to the 16 NSp is a rate-limiting step in viral replication; thus, it is obvious that targeting viral proteases could achieve significant antiviral activity.

2.4.1.2.1 Inhibition of SARS-CoV-2 main protease (Mpro, also called 3CLpro)

Mpro is one of the best characterized drug targets among coronaviruses. This enzyme is essential for processing the translated polyproteins from the viral RNA.

The Mpro works at not less than 11 cleavage sites on the large polyprotein 1ab (replicase 1ab, ~790 kDa); the recognition sequence at most sites is Leu-Gln↓(Ser,Ala,Gly).

The viral replication could be blocked by Mpro inhibitors [65–67]. There are no human proteases with a similar cleavage specificity. Therefore, these inhibitors are not supposed to be toxic. Peptidomimetic alpha keto-amides were reported to be potential Mpro inhibitors [68]. The natural α-keto amides such as eurystatin A and B, complestatin, and aplidine display prolyl endopeptidase inhibitor, HIV replication inhibitor, and antitumor activity, respectively [68]. Also, theaflavin-3,3′-digallate was reported as natural protease inhibitor in SARS-CoV [9]. Other flavonoids are reported to strongly block Mpro activity such as pectolinarin, rhoifolin, herbacetin [69].

2.4.1.2.2 Inhibition of SARS-CoV-2 papain-like protease (PLpro)

PLpro has dual function, beside its role in release of other nonstructural protein, it neutralizes the immune response by the host cell due its deubiquitinating activity, so its inhibition will not only stop the replication cascade but will help the immune system to regain the ability to recognize and destroy the virus [70, 71]. Hirsutenone, a diarylheptanoid from *Alnus Japonica*, was able to inhibit Plpro in uncompetitive manner at IC_{50} = 4.1 μM, which was attributed to the presence of catechol ring and alpha-beta unsaturated ketone [72]. Also tanshinone IIA achieved significant inhibition at IC_{50} = 0.8 μM, the binding of this compound with PLpro was noticed to increase with time indicating the possibility of covalent bond inhibition [73]. Tomentin E geranylated flavonoid was discovered to be mixed-type inhibitor of this target by bio-guided isolation, its IC_{50} = 5.0 μM. The inhibition assay demonstrated that flavonoid bearing dihydropyran ring might be superior inhibitor in comparison to parent compounds. **Figure 5** shows chemical structure of SARS-COV proteases inhibitor from natural products [74].

2.4.1.3 Inhibition of viral replication

After the transcription of viral RNA to the required structural protein, the hijack of the host cell continues to make many replicas of the viral RNA that will be packed

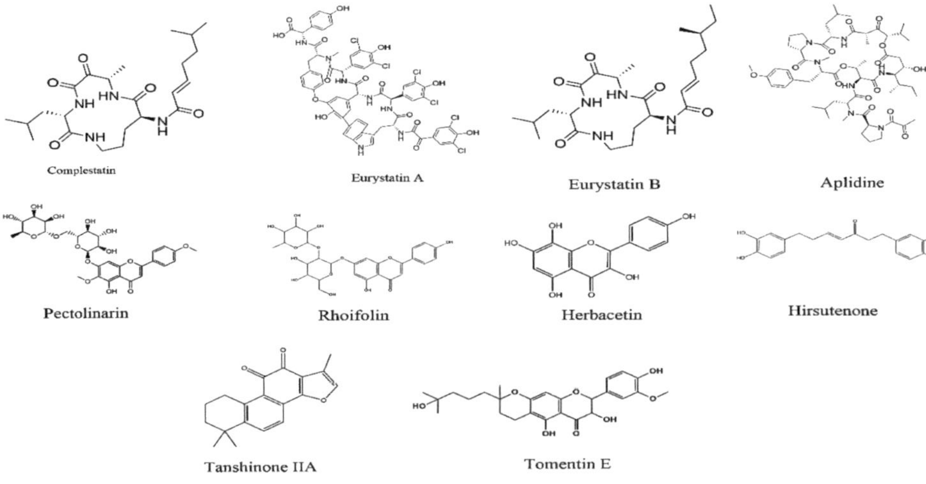

Figure 5.
Chemical structure of natural compounds that inhibit viral proteases (Mpro and PLpro).

and released. The new virus, RNA helicase was found to be crucial to viral genome replication, which explains why it is a potential target for antiviral drug development. Scutellarin inhibits 90% of SARS-COV RNA helicase activity at 10 μM probably by binding to the ADP active site, myricetin showed the same activity but with much lower extent [75]. Interestingly, ivermectin has shown the ability to inhibit RNA helicase of flavivirus [76], taking in consideration that helicase are structurally conservative among most of the viruses. Ivermectin might also be able to exert the same activity in COVID-19, which in fact may explain the potent antiviral activity addressed previously. **Figure 6** shows the chemical structure of the natural helicase inhibitor.

2.4.1.4 The role of natural products in immunity modulation and alleviation of inflammation associated with COVID-19

One of the hallmarks of late-phase COVID-19 infection is uncontrolled intense release of proinflammatory mediators, which is known as cytokines storm. Different types of viruses tend to activate mitogen-activated protein kinase (MAPKs) cascades, which control proliferation and inflammation in order to stimulate the replication process of the virus RNA. Since the upregulation of MAPKs was linked to several inflammatory and autoimmune diseases, it can lead to multiorgan failure and potentially death.

Clinically, in some patients, it has been reported that their immune response to the SARS-CoV-2 virus results in the increase of cytokines IL-6 and IL-10 [77].

Both hydroxychloroquine and chloroquine have immunomodulatory effects and can suppress the increase of immune factors. Bearing this in mind, it is possible that early treatment with either of the drugs may help prevent the progression of the disease to a critical, life-threatening state. In critically ill SARS-CoV-2-infected patients, the use of corticosteroids may be harmful. While the use of immunosuppressants (e.g., tocilizumab) is not ideal either as it can suppress the immune system and lead to an increased risk of infection. In this setting, hydroxychloroquine may be an ideal drug to treat SARS-CoV-2 infection as it can inhibit the virus via its antiviral effects and help mediate the cytokine storm via its immunomodulatory effects [78].

Fortunately, natural products could serve as the perfect solution in such case as they would not only work as antiviral agents but also could help to downregulate proinflammatory gene and protein expression via affecting a plethora of MAPKs and transcriptional factors. LPS-induced expression of proinflammatory cytokine could be considered as an excellent model for screening, since LPS also activates the inflammatory mediators through several pathways.

For example, diarylheptanoids, flavonoids, and triterpenes, which possess antiviral activity as mentioned earlier, were able to suppress the gene expression of TNF-alpha,

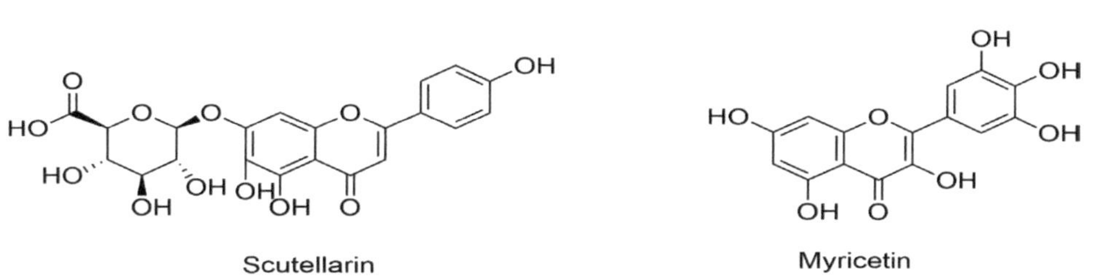

Figure 6.
Chemical structure of the natural helicase inhibitors.

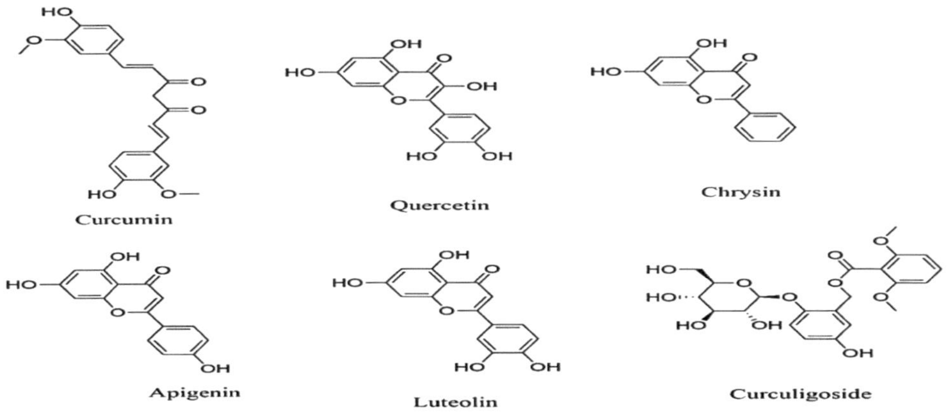

Figure 7.
Chemical structures for the potential natural immunomodulators for cytokine storm associated with COVID-19 infection.

IL-1β, IL-6 in different types of cells such as macrophages and HepG2 induced by LPS by modulating multiple intracellular signaling pathways in macrophages and prevent LPS-induced IL-6 production by reducing the mRNA stability via inhibiting ERK1/2 activation. This could be achieved by natural compounds such as flavokawain A, curcumin, quercetin curculigoside, syringic acid or vanillic acid, licochalcone A, chrysin, apigenin, and luteolin at transcriptional level [78, 79]. In brief, the anti-inflammatory effect of natural products is so prominent to be summarized in this chapter, and they can contribute significantly at reducing the mortality rates associated with COVID-19 complications (**Figure 7**).

3. Artificial intelligence (AI) and machine learning (ML) technologies in drug discovery, diagnosis, and health care of COVID-19

3.1 Drug discovery

Therapeutics: AI and ML in treatment discovery development and/or drug repurposing for COVID-19 based on:

- EHR data and clinical guidelines
- Interaction of human-AI in robotic surgery
- Pharmacogenomics for directing the management of medications

AI may contribute to the advancement of resources to support doctors and ultimately enhance medical outcomes. Fuzzy logic can be used in decision support systems to replicate patient decision-making processes [80–82]. Admittedly, machine learning applied is to clinical data that are regularly collected will produce new knowledge and potentially new perspectives that clinicians lack.

Drug repurposing is hoped to offer a way to establish COVID-19 avoidance and cure policies. For instance, the researchers built a DL approach to classifying current and mercantile medicines for "drug-repurposing," i.e., identifying a quick treatment using existing medicines that can be introduced to patients immediately. The idea that recently created treatment typically needs years to succeed is reviewed before getting to the public motivates research. Although the results are not accepted clinically, new approaches to combat COVID-19 disease are already opening up [83]. In silico medicine is suggested in [84] using the deep generative model to explore drugs (identifying new medicines). This analysis may be used for simulations and computer modeling to obtain compounds for COVID-19 coronavirus by new molecular entities.

IBM reported that it is now offering an analysis service based on the cloud using the COVID-19 dataset that has been educated [85]. Besides, IBM has implemented its proposed drug discovery AI technology, in which 3000 novel COVID-19 molecules have been produced [86]. In the year 2020, a systematic analysis was developed by Zeng et al. [87] to find drugs for COVID-19. With the support of active Amazon Web Services (AWS), a DL-based model was developed, and 41 data on drug types were validated. As for performance metrics, true-positive rate (TPR), false-positive rate (FPR), etc., have been presented, and the approach suggested by the author is explicit that DL serves as an important instrument for exploring therapeutics.

3.2 Diagnostics

Earlier, our research team had presented the usefulness of AI and ML in diagnosis of several diseases [88–90]. However, COVID-19 diagnosis was based on AI.

- Multiomics and clinical data

- Records of Electronic Health (HER) data and expert knowledge

3.2.1 Image data and deep learning

Nour et al. [91] have developed a DL model for COVID-19 detection, as CNN is applied as a feature extractor. For performance assessment, chest X-ray images dataset is taken into account. For feeding ML methods such as K-nearest neighbour (KNN), Decision Tree (DT), and *support vector machines* (SVM), the deep feature that has been extracted with the aid of CNN is utilized. Precision, F-score, etc., are used as output variables. Among other suggested approaches, SVM yields greater precision.

Pereira et al. [92] proposed a new model for forecasting the dynamics of COVID-19 that have cases that have happened in other countries or places with similar emission patterns. For all subregions and accessible countries, they implemented a grouping algorithm.

3.3 Health care

Big data in the administration of hospitals, epidemiology, insurance, medication interactions and complications, outcomes reviews based on quality, epidemic tracking.

Speech datasets include breath sounds and cough, which can be utilized for COVID-19 diagnoses and its prediction for illness seriousness. Machine learning, statistical techniques, and big data may be used to the datasets for prediction functions about the disease. Various open-source datasets for COVID-19 included mobility, diagnosis, contagion assessment, NPI analysis, statistic relationships, and sentiment analysis.

4. Concluding remarks and future perspective

COVID-19 causes a gigantic load to the healthcare system, particularly in patients with preexisting conditions comorbidities. A comprehensive study is presented about COVID-19 symptoms, clinical classification (mild, moderate, severe, critical cases), and the risk indicators for COVID-19 infection with comorbidities.

Natural products (NPs) have been used for centuries for treatments of different maladies and inspired scientists to develop safer and more effective drugs. The COVID-19 is complex clinical condition that comprises inflammatory components. Although selective inhibitor could be developed for inhibiting critical molecular target in the life of cycle, compounds with multitargeting activity may be more favorable to reduce the possibility of mutation development. Optimum drug should be able to modulate host cell and viral-related mechanisms. This is where natural products could play important role since their ability to bind effectively to targets with completely different homology. Nevertheless, the anti-inflammatory attribute of NPs is another advantage that should be considered during choosing therapeutic protocol. Finally, the observed antiviral activity of different phytochemicals should initiate repurposing campaign of untested NPs to identify new antiviral compounds, which could be exploited to design more effective drugs with optimum pharmacokinetic properties. This study presents briefly the value of AI and ML as powerful tools in healthcare, clinical, drug industry, diagnosis, decision-making, and improvement of the selection criteria for the most appropriate protocol for the treatment of COVID-19.

Acknowledgements

The author would like to thank Ms. Rowida Omar (Department of Pharmacognosy, Faculty of Pharmacy, Delta University, Gamsa, Egypt) and Mr. Abdullah A. Elgazar (Department of Pharmacognosy, Faculty of Pharmacy, Kafrelsheikh University, Egypt) for their great efforts in providing valuable materials of the first draft and Mrs. Zahraa Tarek (Computer Science Department, Faculty of Computer and Information, Mansoura University, Egypt) for providing materials on artificial intelligence section.

Conflict of interest

The authors declare no conflict of interest.

Author details

Farid A. Badria
Faculty of Pharmacy, Department of Pharmacognosy, Mansoura University, Mansoura, Egypt

*Address all correspondence to: badri002@mans.edu.eg

References

[1] Su S, Wong G, Shi W, Liu J, Lai AC, Zhou J, et al. Epidemiology, genetic recombination, and pathogenesis of coronaviruses. Trends in Microbiology. 2016;**24**(6):490-502

[2] Hoffmann M, Kleine-Weber H, Schroeder S, Krüger N, Herrler T, Erichsen S, et al. SARS-CoV-2 cell entry depends on ACE2 and TMPRSS2 and is blocked by a clinically proven protease inhibitor. Cell. 2020;**181**:271-280

[3] Yang N, Shen H-M. Targeting the endocytic pathway and autophagy process as a novel therapeutic strategy in COVID-19. International Journal of Biological Sciences. 2020;**16**(10):1724-1731

[4] Inoue Y, Tanaka N, Tanaka Y, Inoue S, Morita K, Zhuang M, et al. Clathrin-dependent entry of severe acute respiratory syndrome coronavirus into target cells expressing ACE2 with the cytoplasmic tail deleted. Journal of Virology. 2007;**81**(16):8722-8729

[5] Huang IC, Bosch BJ, Li F, Li W, Lee KH, Ghiran S, et al. SARS coronavirus, but not human coronavirus NL63, utilizes cathepsin L to infect ACE2-expressing cells. The Journal of Biological Chemistry. 2006;**281**(6):3198-3203

[6] Simmons G, Gosalia DN, Rennekamp AJ, Reeves JD, Diamond SL, Bates P. Inhibitors of cathepsin L prevent severe acute respiratory syndrome coronavirus entry. Proceedings of the National Academy of Sciences of the United States of America. 2005;**102**(33):11876-11881

[7] Mathew C, Ghildyal R. CRM1 inhibitors for antiviral therapy. Frontiers in Microbiology. 2017;**8**:1171

[8] Cui J, Li F, Shi Z-L. Origin and evolution of pathogenic coronaviruses. Nature Reviews Microbiology. 2019;**17**(3):181-192

[9] Báez-Santos YM, St John SE, Mesecar AD. The SARS-coronavirus papain-like protease: Structure, function and inhibition by designed antiviral compounds. Antiviral Research. 2015;**115**:21-38

[10] Liu C, Zhou Q, Li Y, Garner LV, Watkins SP, Carter LJ, et al. Research and Development on Therapeutic Agents and Vaccines for COVID-19 and Related Human Coronavirus Diseases. Washington, D.C., USA: ACS Publications; 2020

[11] Keum Y-S, Jeong Y-J. Development of chemical inhibitors of the SARS coronavirus: Viral helicase as a potential target. Biochemical Pharmacology. 2012;**84**(10):1351-1358

[12] Masters PS. The molecular biology of coronaviruses. Advances in Virus Research. 2006;**66**:193-292

[13] Fung TS, Liu DX. Human coronavirus: Host-pathogen interaction. Annual Review of Microbiology. 2019;**73**:529-557

[14] Amanat F, Krammer F. SARS-CoV-2 vaccines: Status report. Immunity. 2020:583-589

[15] Khalili M, Karamouzian M, Nasiri N, Javadi S, Mirzazadeh A, Sharifi H. Epidemiological characteristics of COVID-19: A systemic review and meta-analysis. MedRxiv. 2020;**148**:1-7

[16] Available from: https://www.who.int/news-room/questions-and-answers/

item/coronavirus-disease-(covid-19) vaccines?

[17] Xavier AR, Silva JS, Almeida JPC, Conceição JFF, Lacerda GS, Kanaan S. COVID-19: Clinical and laboratory manifestations in novel coronavirus infection. Jornal Brasileiro de Patologia e Medicina Laboratorial. 2020;**56**

[18] He S, Tang S, Rong L. A discrete stochastic model of the COVID-19 outbreak: Forecast and control. Mathematical Biosciences and Engineering. 2020;**17**:2792-2804

[19] Guan W, Ni Z, Hu Y, Liang W, Ou C, He J, et al. Clinical characteristics of coronavirus disease 2019 in China. New England Journal of Medicine. 2020;**382**(18):1708-1720

[20] Li X, Xu Z, Wang T, Xu X, Li H, Sun Q , et al. Clinical laboratory characteristics of severe patients with coronavirus disease 2019 (COVID-19): A systematic review and meta-analysis. Clinical Epidemiology and Global Health. 2020

[21] Liang JJ, Liu J, Chen Y, Ye B, Li N, Wang X, et al. Characteristics of laboratory findings of COVID-19 patients with comorbid diabetes mellitus. Diabetes Research and Clinical Practice. 2020;**167**(108351):1-5

[22] Brooks SK, Webster RK, Smith LE, Woodland L, Wessely S, Greenberg N, et al. The psychological impact of quarantine and how to reduce it: Rapid review of the evidence. The Lancet. 2020;**395**(10227):912-920

[23] Wu J, Wu X, Zeng W, Guo D, Fang Z, Chen L, et al. Chest CT findings in patients with coronavirus disease 2019 and its relationship with clinical features. Investigative Radiology. 2020;**55**(5):257

[24] Wang K, Kang S, Tian R, Zhang X, Wang Y. Imaging manifestations and diagnostic value of chest CT of coronavirus disease 2019 (COVID-19) in the Xiaogan area. Clinical Radiology. 2020;**75**(5):341-347

[25] Yang W, Cao Q, Qin L, Wang X, Cheng Z, Pan A, et al. Clinical characteristics and imaging manifestations of the 2019 novel coronavirus disease (COVID-19): A multi-center study in Wenzhou city, Zhejiang, China. Journal of Infection. 2020;**80**(4):388-393

[26] Li K, Fang Y, Li W, Pan C, Qin P, Zhong Y, et al. CT image visual quantitative evaluation and clinical classification of coronavirus disease (COVID-19). European Radiology. 2020:1-10

[27] Wang M, Cao R, Zhang L, Yang X, Liu J, Xu M, et al. Remdesivir and chloroquine effectively inhibit the recently emerged novel coronavirus (2019-nCoV) in vitro. Cell Research. 2020;**30**(3):269-271

[28] Jun C, Yun L, Xiuhong X, Ping L, Feng L, Tao L, et al. Efficacies of lopinavir/ritonavir and abidol in the treatment of novel coronavirus pneumonia. Chinese Journal of Infectious Diseases. 2020:E008-E008

[29] Zumla A, Hui DS, Azhar EI, Memish ZA, Maeurer M. Reducing mortality from 2019-nCoV: Host-directed therapies should be an option. The Lancet. 2020;**395**(10224): e35-e36

[30] Mair-Jenkins J, Saavedra-Campos M, Baillie JK, Cleary P, Khaw F-M, Lim WS, et al. The effectiveness of convalescent plasma and hyperimmune immunoglobulin for the treatment of severe acute respiratory infections of viral etiology: A systematic review and exploratory meta-analysis. The Journal of Infectious Diseases. 2015;**211**(1):80-90

[31] Chen Q, Wang L, Xie M, Li X, Recommendations for Influenza, Streptococcus pneumoniae Vaccination in Elderly People in China Writing Group, Geriatric Respiratory Group and Chinese Society of Geriatrics. Recommendations for influenza and Streptococcus pneumoniae vaccination in elderly people in China. Aging Medicine. 2020;**3**(1):4-14

[32] Badria FA, (Ed.). Drug Repurposing—Hypothesis, Molecular Aspects and Therapeutic Applications. London, UK: IntechOpen; 2020. DOI: 10.5772/intechopen.83082

[33] Badria F, Fayed HA, Ibraheem AK, Mazyed EA. Formulation of sodium valproate nanospanlastics as a promising approach for drug repurposing in the treatment of androgenic alopecia. Pharmaceutics. 2020;**12**(9):866

[34] Badria F, Elgazar A. Drug repurposing in dermatology: Molecular biology and omics approach. In: Badria F, editor. Drug Repurposing: Hypothesis, Molecular Aspects and Therapeutic Applications. London: IntechOpen; 2020. DOI: 10.5772/intechopen.93344

[35] El-Mesery M, Seher A, El-Shafey M, El-Dosoky M, Badria FA. Repurposing of quinoline alkaloids identifies their ability to enhance doxorubicin-induced sub-G0/G1 phase cell cycle arrest and apoptosis in cervical and hepatocellular. Biotechnology and Applied Biochemistry. 2021;**68**(4):832-840

[36] Ibrahim MG, El-Senduny FF, Youssef MM, Elimam DM, Bar FMA. Acetyl glycyrrhetinic acid methyl ester as a promising glycyrrhizin derivative against the breast cancer cells (MCF-7). Journal of Reports in Pharmaceutical Sciences. 2019;**8**(2):161

[37] El-Senduny FF, Zidane MM, Youssef MM, Badria FA. An approach to treatment of liver cancer by novel glycyrrhizin derivative. Anti-Cancer Agents in Medicinal Chemistry. 2019;**19**(15):1863-1873

[38] Bar FMA, Elimam DM, Mira AS, El-Senduny FF, Badria FA. Derivatization, molecular docking and *in vitro* acetylcholinesterase inhibitory activity of glycyrrhizin as a selective anti-Alzheimer agent. Natural Product Research. 2019;**33**(18):2591-2599

[39] Wang Y, Chen L. Tissue distributions of antiviral drugs affect their capabilities of reducing viral loads in COVID-19 treatment. European Journal of Pharmacology. 2020;**889**:173634

[40] Ye C, Gao M, Lin W, Yu K, Li P, Chen G. Theoretical study of the anti-NCP molecular mechanism of traditional Chinese Medicine Lianhua-Qingwen Formula (LQF). Polar. 2020;**2**(21.52):10-68

[41] Wu H, Wang J, Yang Y, Li T, Cao Y, Qu Y, et al. Preliminary exploration of the mechanism of Qingfei Paidu decoction against novel coronavirus pneumonia based on network pharmacology and molecular docking technology. Acta Pharmaceutica Sinica. 2020;**55**:374-383

[42] Xu D, Xu Y, Wang Z, Lv Y, Zhu H, Song T. Mechanism of Qingfeipaidu decoction on COVID-19 based on network pharmacology. Pharmacol Clin Chin Materia. 2020;**158**(104939):1-11

[43] Fan J-X, Qin X-M, Li Z-Y. Mechanism of Farfarae Flos in Qingfei Paidu Decoction against COVID-19 based on network pharmacology and molecular docking. Chinese Traditional and Herbal Drugs. 2020;**11**:2317-2325

[44] Huang YF, Bai C, He F, Xie Y, Zhou H. Review on the potential action

mechanisms of Chinese medicines in treating coronavirus disease 2019 (COVID-19). Pharmacological Research. 2020;**158**:104939. DOI: 10.1016/j.phrs.2020.104939

[45] Deng YJ, Liu BW, He ZX, Liu T, Zheng RL, Di Yang A, et al. Study on active compounds from Huoxiang Zhengqi oral liquid for prevention of coronavirus disease 2019 (COVID-19) based on network pharmacology and molecular docking. Chinese Traditional and Herbal Drugs. 2020;**51**(5):1113-1122

[46] Shi Y, Wei J, Liu M, Jin X, Zhou H, Zhu W, et al. Study on the overall regulation of Xuebijing injection in treating corona virus disease 2019. Shanghai Journal of Traditional Chinese Medicine. 2020;**54**:1-7

[47] Jimilihan S et al. Study on the active components in the adjuvant treatment of novel coronavirus pneumonia (COVID-19) with Jinhua Qinggan Granules based on network pharmacology and molecular docking. Journal of Chinese Medicinal Materials. 2020;**225**:1-10

[48] Glende J, Schwegmann-Wessels C, Al-Falah M, Pfefferle S, Qu X, Deng H, et al. Importance of cholesterol-rich membrane microdomains in the interaction of the S protein of SARS-coronavirus with the cellular receptor angiotensin-converting enzyme 2. Virology. 2008;**381**(2):215-221

[49] Heaton NS, Randall G. Multifaceted roles for lipids in viral infection. Trends in Microbiology. 2011;**19**(7):368-375

[50] Guo H, Huang M, Yuan Q, Wei Y, Gao Y, Mao L, et al. The important role of lipid raft-mediated attachment in the infection of cultured cells by coronavirus infectious bronchitis virus *Beaudette* strain. PLoS One. 2017;**12**(1):e0170123. DOI: 10.1371/journal.pone.0170123

[51] Baglivo M, Baronio M, Natalini G, Beccari T, Chiurazzi P, Fulcheri E, et al. Natural small molecules as inhibitors of coronavirus lipid-dependent attachment to host cells: A possible strategy for reducing SARS-COV-2 infectivity? Acta Bio-medica: Atenei Parmensis. 2020;**91**(1):161

[52] Andrade PB, Valentão P, Pereira DM, editors. Natural Products Targeting Clinically Relevant Enzymes. 3rd ed. Hoboken, New Jersey, U.S: Wiley Online Library; 2017. ISBN: 978-3-527-34205-1

[53] de Haan CA, Rottier PJ. Molecular interactions in the assembly of coronaviruses. Advances in Virus Research. 2005;**64**:165-230

[54] Devaux CA, Rolain J-M, Colson P, Raoult D. New insights on the antiviral effects of chloroquine against coronavirus: What to expect for COVID-19? International Journal of Antimicrobial Agents. 2020;**55**(5):105938:1-6

[55] Yang Z-Y, Huang Y, Ganesh L, Leung K, Kong W-P, Schwartz O, et al. pH-dependent entry of severe acute respiratory syndrome coronavirus is mediated by the spike glycoprotein and enhanced by dendritic cell transfer through DC-SIGN. Journal of Virology. 2004;**78**(11):5642-5650

[56] Vidal-Albalat A, González FV. Chapter 6—Natural products as cathepsin inhibitors. In: Atta ur R, editor. Studies in Natural Products Chemistry. Vol. 50. Amsterdam, The Netherlands: Elsevier; 2016. pp. 179-213

[57] Burkard C, Verheije MH, Haagmans BL, van Kuppeveld FJ, Rottier PJ, Bosch BJ, et al. ATP1A1-mediated Src signaling inhibits coronavirus entry into host cells. Journal of Virology. 2015;**89**(8):4434-4448

[58] Jeon S, Ko M, Lee J, Choi I, Byun SY, Park S, et al. Identification of antiviral drug candidates against SARS-CoV-2 from FDA-approved drugs. bioRxiv. 2020.03.20.999730. 2020:480-485

[59] Margarucci L, Monti MC, Fontanella B, Riccio R, Casapullo A. Chemical proteomics reveals bolinaquinone as a clathrin-mediated endocytosis inhibitor. Molecular Biosystems. 2011;7(2):480-485

[60] Elkin SR, Oswald NW, Reed DK, Mettlen M, MacMillan JB, Schmid SL. Ikarugamycin: A natural product inhibitor of clathrin-mediated endocytosis. Traffic (Copenhagen, Denmark). 2016;**17**(10):1139-1149

[61] Caly L, Druce JD, Catton MG, Jans DA, Wagstaff KM. The FDA-approved drug ivermectin inhibits the replication of SARS- CoV-2 in vitro. Antiviral Research. 2020;**178**:104787-104803

[62] Yang SNY, Atkinson SC, Wang C, Lee A, Bogoyevitch MA, Borg NA, et al. The broad spectrum antiviral ivermectin targets the host nuclear transport importin α/β1 heterodimer. Antiviral Research. 2020;**177**:104760

[63] Hilgenfeld R. From SARS to MERS: Crystallographic studies on coronaviral proteases enable antiviral drug design. The FEBS Journal. 2014;**281**(18):4085-4096

[64] García-Fernández R, Ziegelmüller P, González L, Mansur M, Machado Y, Redecke L, et al. Two variants of the major serine protease inhibitor from the sea anemone Stichodactyla helianthus, expressed in *Pichia pastoris*. Protein Expression and Purification. 2016;**123**:42-50

[65] Zhang L, Lin D, Sun X, Curth U, Drosten C, Sauerhering L, et al. Crystal structure of SARS-CoV-2 main protease provides a basis for design of improved α-ketoamide inhibitors. Science. 2020;**368**(6489):409-412

[66] Muthukumar A, Sangeetha S, Sekar G. Recent developments in functionalization of acyclic α-keto amides. Organic & Biomolecular Chemistry. 2018;**16**(39):7068-7083

[67] Chen C-N, Lin CPC, Huang K-K, Chen W-C, Hsieh H-P, Liang P-H, et al. Inhibition of SARS-CoV 3C-like protease activity by Theaflavin-3,3′-digallate (TF3). Evidence-based Complementary and Alternative Medicine. 2005;**2**(2): 209-215

[68] Jo S, Kim S, Shin DH, Kim M-S. Inhibition of SARS-CoV 3CL protease by flavonoids. Journal of Enzyme Inhibition and Medicinal Chemistry. 2020;**35**(1):145-151

[69] Barretto N, Jukneliene D, Ratia K, Chen Z, Mesecar AD, Baker SC. The papain-like protease of severe acute respiratory syndrome coronavirus has deubiquitinating activity. Journal of Virology. 2005;**79**(24):15189-15198

[70] Park J-Y, Jae Jeong H, Hoon Kim J, Min Kim Y, Park S-J, Kim D, et al. Diarylheptanoids from Alnus japonica inhibit papain-like protease of severe acute respiratory syndrome coronavirus. Biological & Pharmaceutical Bulletin. 2012;**35**(11):2036-2042

[71] Park J-Y, Kim JH, Kim YM, Jeong HJ, Kim DW, Park KH, et al. Tanshinones as selective and slow-binding inhibitors for SARS-CoV cysteine proteases. Bioorganic & Medicinal Chemistry. 2012;**20**(19):5928-5935

[72] Cho JK, Curtis-Long MJ, Lee KH, Kim DW, Ryu HW, Yuk HJ, et al. Geranylated flavonoids displaying

SARS-CoV papain-like protease inhibition from the fruits of Paulownia tomentosa. Bioorganic & Medicinal Chemistry. 2013;**21**(11):3051-3057

[73] Yu M-S, Lee J, Lee JM, Kim Y, Chin Y-W, Jee J-G, et al. Identification of myricetin and scutellarein as novel chemical inhibitors of the SARS coronavirus helicase, nsP13. Bioorganic & Medicinal Chemistry Letters. 2012;**22**(12):4049-4054

[74] Mastrangelo E, Pezzullo M, De Burghgraeve T, Kaptein S, Pastorino B, Dallmeier K, et al. Ivermectin is a potent inhibitor of flavivirus replication specifically targeting NS3 helicase activity: New prospects for an old drug. Journal of Antimicrobial Chemotherapy. 2012;**67**(8):1884-1894

[75] Huang C, Wang Y, Li X, Ren L, Zhao J, Hu Y, et al. Clinical features of patients infected with 2019 novel coronavirus in Wuhan, China. The Lancet. 2020;**395**(10223):497-506

[76] Yao X, Ye F, Zhang M, Cui C, Huang B, Niu P, et al. In vitro antiviral activity and projection of optimized dosing design of hydroxychloroquine for the treatment of severe acute respiratory syndrome coronavirus 2 (SARS-CoV-2). Clinical Infectious Diseases. 2020;**71**(15):732-739

[77] Grigore A. Plant phenolic compounds as immunomodulatory agents. In: Phenolic Compounds–Biological Activity. London, UK: IntechOpen; 2017. pp. 75-98

[78] Badria FA, Abdelaziz EA, Hassan AH, Elgazar AE, Mazyed EA. Development of provesicular nanodelivery system of curcumin as a safe and effective antiviral agent: Statistical optimization, in vitro characterization, and antiviral effectiveness. Molecules. 2020;**25**(23):5668

[79] Badria F, Mazyed E. Formulation of nanospanlastics as a promising approach for improving the topical delivery of a natural leukotriene inhibitor (3-Acetyl-11-keto-β-Boswellic acid): Statistical optimization, in vitro characterization, and ex vivo permeation study. Drug Design, Development and Therapy. 2020;**14**:3697-3721

[80] Elmogy M, Elfetouh A, Elhefny M, Badria F. Foorc: A fuzzy ontology-based representation for obesity related cancer knowledge, Ain Shams University, Faculty of Computer and Information Science. IJIC1S. 2016;**6**(3):15-32

[81] Elhefny MA, Elmogy M, Elfetouh AA, Badria FA. Developing a fuzzy OWL ontology for obesity related cancer domain. International Journal of Medical Engineering and Informatics. 2017;**9**(2):162-187

[82] Shoaip N, Elmogy M, Riad AM, Badria FA. Missing data treatment using interval-valued fuzzy rough sets with svm. International Journal of Advancements in Computing Technology. 2015;**7**(5):37

[83] Beck BR, Shin B, Choi Y, Park S, Kang K. Predicting commercially available antiviral drugs that may act on the novel coronavirus (SARS-CoV-2) through a drug-target interaction deep learning model. Computational and Structural Biotechnology Journal. 2020;**18**:784-790

[84] Zhavoronkov A, Aladinskiy V, Zhebrak A, Zagribelnyy B, Terentiev V, Bezrukov DS, et al. Potential COVID-2019 3C-like protease inhibitors designed using generative deep learning approaches. Insilico Medicine Hong Kong Ltd A. 2020;**307**:E1

[85] A I F A et al. COVID-19 Open Research Dataset Challenge (CORD-19):

An AI Challenge with AI2, CZI, MSR, Georgetown, NIH & The White House. USA: Kaggle; 2020

[86] Gil D. IBM releases novel AI-powered technologies to help health and research community accelerate the discovery of medical insights and treatments for COVID-19. IBM. 2020

[87] Zeng X, Song X, Ma T, Pan X, Zhou Y, Hou Y, et al. Repurpose open data to discover therapeutics for COVID-19 using deep learning. Journal of Proteome Research. 2020;**19**(11):4624-4636

[88] Badria FA, Shoaip N, Elmogy M, Riad AM, Zaghlou H. In: Hassanien AE, Tolba MF, Taher AA, editors. A framework for ovarian cancer diagnosis based on amino acids using fuzzyrough sets with SVM, Advanced Machine Learning Technologies and Applications. AMLTA 2014. Communications in Computer and Information Science. Vol. 488. Cham: Springer; 2014. pp. 389-400

[89] Sweidan S, El-Sappagh S, El-Bakry H, Sabbeh S, Badria FA, Kwak KS. A fibrosis diagnosis clinical decision support system using fuzzy knowledge. Arabian Journal for Science and Engineering. 2019;**44**(4):3781-3800

[90] Shoaip N, Elmogy MM, Riad AM, Zaghloul H, Badria FA. Early-stage ovarian cancer diagnosis using fuzzy rough sets with SVM classification. In: Handbook of Research on Machine Learning Innovations and Trends. Vol. 43-60. 2017

[91] Nour M, Cömert Z, Polat K. A novel medical diagnosis model for COVID-19 infection detection based on deep features and Bayesian optimization. Applied Soft Computing. 2020;**97**:106580

[92] Pereira I, Guérin J, Junior A, Garcia G, Piscitelli P, Miani A, et al. Forecasting Covid-19 dynamics in Brazil: A data driven approach. International Journal of Environmental Research and Public Health. 2020;**17**:5115

Chapter 3

Antiviral Drugs and Their Roles in the Treatment of Coronavirus Infection

Radi Alsafi, Saad Alghamdi and Mohammad Asif

Abstract

Viruses are the major pathogenic agents that cause various diseases. Antiviral drugs are used for the treatment of viral infections. Emergent advances of antiviral drugs are focused on two different approaches: targeting the host cell factors or the viruses themselves. Antiviral drugs that directly target the viruses include virus entry inhibitors, virus attachment inhibitors, uncoating inhibitors, protease inhibitors, polymerase inhibitors, nucleoside inhibitors, integrase inhibitors, and nucleotide reverse transcriptase. The protease inhibitors, viral DNA polymerase, and integrase inhibitors are the most commonly used antiviral drugs. Still, there are no effective antiviral drugs existing for several viral infections. Coronavirus disease-2019 (COVID-19) or SARS-CoV-2 is the newest member of the coronavirus family. No specific drugs particularly antiviral drugs have been approved for the treatment of COVID-19. Thus, it is extremely crucial to identify new drugs for the treatment of the COVID-19 outbreak. Various antiviral drugs are used for COVID-19 treatment. Currently, various drugs are under investigation to treat COVID-19 patients. Promising clinical outcomes for COVID-19 can be obtained by using alpha-interferon, remdesivir, lopinavir-ritonavir, favipiravir, ribavirin, umifenovir, oseltamivir, etc. Here, we reviewed anti-COVID-19 potencies of currently available antiviral drugs, and some antiviral drugs have been effective or prevent the spread of coronavirus.

Keywords: antiviral drugs, SARS-CoV-2, drug discovery, mechanism of action, pandemic

1. Introduction

Coronaviruses (CoVs) belong to the subfamily Orthocoronavirinae in the family of Coronaviridae. In this family, there are four types of viruses: α-coronavirus, β-coronavirus, γ-coronavirus, δ-coronavirus [1]. The CoV genome is an enveloped, positive-sense, and single-stranded RNA, and it has the largest genome of known RNA viruses. It is known that α- and β-CoV types cause infections in mammals as δ- and γ-CoVs infect birds [2]. Severe acute respiratory syndrome (SARS) and the Middle East respiratory syndrome (MERS) belonging to β-CoVs are the most aggressive strains of coronaviruses and cause viral pneumonia outbreaks [3, 4]. SARS-CoV disease is a kind of pneumonia and caused by novel CoV whose genome structure was more than 82% identical to those of SARS-CoV, named coronavirus disease 2019 (COVID-19) [5, 6]. SARS-Cov-2 is a beta gene virus genetically very close to bat-CoVRaTG13, and bat-SL-CoVZC45 Covs can cause severe illness. As the COVID-19 outbreak turned into a global threat, the World Health Organization (WHO) announced it as a global pandemic on 12 March 2020. The COVID-19 pandemic has changed the scenario of the entire world. COVID-19 outbreak started in Wuhan, China, has globally spread to 219 countries and territories [7]. Currently, there are few vaccines for COVID-19. Their acceptance and efficacy are an issue of debate across the whole world. Therefore, there is an urgent need to find drugs or vaccines for the treatment of COVID-19 infections effectively. However, there are some studies related to the use of known drugs such as remdesivir and chloroquine that have proved efficacy on COVID-19 infection. We summarize some antiviral drugs as therapeutic options for the treatment of COVID-19 [8].

COVID-19 mainly attacks the respiratory-tract-associated organs. Additionally, the virus has shown impact various to other organs or systems such as the gastrointestinal system, nervous system, etc. [9]. The most common symptoms in COVID-19 patients are fever, dry cough, loss of taste, lethargy, shortness of breath, dyspnea, chest pain, fatigue, myalgia, whereas headache, dizziness, abdominal pain, diarrhea, nausea, and vomiting are less commonly observed [10, 11]. Anosmia is also one of the most critical symptoms in COVID-19 patients [12]. COVID-19 is more contagious than other coronaviruses, and its transmission rate is higher than the closely related strain, SARS-CoV-10 [13]. Currently, new variants of COVID-19 are reported from different regions of the world. Coronavirus interacts with cell surface receptors such as angiotensin-converting enzyme-2 (ACE-2) and neuropilin to gain entry inside the cell. The receptor-binding domain of viral spike protein is essential in SARS-CoV-2 entry into the host cell via surface ACE-2 [14]. Recently, another cell receptor Neuropilin-1 was found to be involved in SARS-CoV-2 entry. After binding to the receptor, the conformational change in the spike protein leads to virus fusion with the host cell membrane. The virus may transfer the RNA directly inside the cells or may proceed through the endosomal pathway [15]. Upon translation of viral RNA, the viral replicase polyprotein PP1a and PP1ab are produced and cleaved into small products by viral endopeptidase [16]. RNA-dependent RNA polymerase (RdRp) produces subgenomic RNAs by discontinuous transcription [16, 17]. This further gets translated into respective viral proteins. After processing through the endoplasmic reticulum (ER), ER-Golgi intermediate compartment (ERGIC), and Golgi complex, the viral RNA and proteins are assembled into virions. These virions are transported through vesicles and exocytosed for transmission. These steps of the viral life cycle are beneficial virus inhibition targets for different drugs. The coronaviruses are ribonucleic acid (RNA) viruses, which have a positive single-strand RNA [14, 18]. When SARS-CoV-2 enters the body and comes in contact with the host cell membrane, some changes occur in the structure of the virus. The human TMPRSS2 protein alters the conformation of the spike glycoprotein in the virus. Two substantial protease enzymes, 3-chymotrypsin-like protease (3CLpro) and papain-like protease (PLPro), have essential roles in its viral replication process after it enters the host cell via ACE2 receptors [19]. The expression of several genes, such as AHCYL2, ZNF385B, etc., appears to have a strong correlation with the expression of ACE2 and TMPRSS2 protein receptors in human healthy and normal lung cells [20].

However, repurposing drugs could prove to be beneficial tactics for finding COVID-19 treatment, including cost-effectiveness, elimination of some clinical trial steps, faster on-field availability, combining the drugs with other possible drugs, and the invention of information about the mechanisms of the existing drug. Researchers were able to develop the possible COVID-19 medications using information from previous CoVs therapies, genetic sequences, and protein modeling studies. Antimalarials, antivirals, antibiotics, and corticosteroids are among the most often studied medications, and they have been repurposed based on their ability to neutralize viruses, reduce lung inflammation, or alleviate other illness symptoms. Chloroquine (CQ), hydroxychloroquine (HCQ), and azithromycin (AZM) are the most often utilized antiviral drugs against COVID-19, since they have already demonstrated reasonable antiviral efficacy against SARS-CoV, MERS-CoV, and SARS-CoV-2. Anti-HIV medications lopinavir/ritonavir (LPV/RTV) are being studied for COVID-19 since they were successful in previous CoV epidemics. Furthermore, the anti-Ebola medicine remdesivir (RDV) was evaluated for COVID-19 and garnered further attention.

Similarly, favipiravir (FPV), ribavirin (RBV), umifenovir (UFV), and oseltamivir (OTV) have broad-spectrum antiviral activities and clinically tested against COVID-19. The effective uses of HCQ, RDV, LPV/RTV, or LPV/RTV in combination with Interferon (IFN) β-1a against COVID-19 [21], all these drugs had little or no effect on overall mortality, initiation of ventilation, and duration of hospital stay in hospitalized patients. So far, to treat severe and critical COVID-19, only corticosteroids have proven effective [21]. Other drugs, such as Angiotensin-Converting-Enzyme inhibitors (ACEi), have also been used to treat COVID-19. However, no clear correlation was reported between mortality rate and ACEi drugs in hypertension patients with COVID-19 [22]. Due to the possibility of secondary infection in these patients, antibiotics have been used as various protocols [23].

Umifenovir (UFV) may interact with SARS-CoV-2 surface glycoproteins and lipids and obstruct the interaction with the entry receptor ACE-2. Antibodies against SARS-CoV-2 may prevent the virus from entering the body and causing illness. Chloroquine (CQ), hydroxychloroquine (HCQ), and azithromycin (AZM) can raise endosomal pH, making viral entrance and RNA release more difficult. CQ, HCQ, and AZM all have immunomodulatory properties. RDV, FPV, and RBV are nucleoside inhibitors that impede RNA replication and reduce RNA-dependent RNA polymerase activity. Fraternization of LPV with viral protease may change proteolysis. OTV may interact with components involved in exocytosis, preventing the virus from leaving the cell. Antibodies against cytokine receptors and corticosteroids have been shown to have anti-inflammatory properties in the face of excessive immune responses. Drugs such as CQ are wide-spectrum inhibitors of viral cell entry, and RDV is a wide-spectrum RNA polymerase inhibitor. SARS-CoV-2 infection concurrently triggers the host immune system and an inflammatory cascade response (cytokine storm). These are being targeted in the treatment of COVID-19 patients [23].

So far, no fully effective drug has been discovered against this virus. The antiviral drugs, usually nucleoside analogs or intracellular proteases, block the virus by preventing its entry into the cell or by interfering with its replication inside the cell. Protease inhibitors target certain proteases, whereas fusion inhibitors block the fusion phase of viral entrance. Transcription inhibitors impede viral replication by inhibiting RNA-dependent RNA polymerase during the reverse transcription process. Nucleoside reverse transcriptases are some of the transcriptase inhibitors. M2 channel protein is a target for certain antivirals. In this chapter, we have provided information about repurposed drugs that are used against COVID-19, the mechanism of activity, therapeutic regimens, pharmacokinetics, and drug-drug interactions [7, 8].

2. SARS-CoV-2 life cycle and potential targets

The rationale major biochemical events and components in the replication cycle of coronavirus are considered as targets for currently developed drugs. These include the spike protein, proteolytic enzymes, and RNA-dependent RNA polymerase [24]. SARS-CoV-2 is transmitted mainly via respiratory droplets. The virus enters the host cells through two pathways, either via endosomes or plasma membrane fusion. In both mechanisms, the viral S protein mediates attachment to the membrane of the host cell and engages ACE2 as the entry receptor [25]. A host protease termed transmembrane serine protease 2 (TMPRSS2) activates the connection between S protein and ACE-2 [26]. S protein is used by the virus to destroy antibodies and make it simpler for it to attach to host receptors [27]. Beta-coronaviruses generally employ hemagglutinin-esterase (HE) to bind to sialic acid on the glycoprotein surface, despite the fact that the fusion machinery of SARS-CoV-2 remains unknown [28]. Fusion inhibitors might be used to prevent these fusion stages.

The envelope is peeled off when fusion is complete, and the SARS-CoV-2 genome, together with its nucleocapsid, penetrates the cytoplasm of the host cell. Its genome comprises the open reading frames 1a and 1b (ORF1a and ORF1b) genes, which create two polyproteins (pp) named pp1a and pp1b, which aid in the viral translation process by hijacking host ribosomes [29]. Main protease (Mpro) and papain-like protease (Ppro) break these polyproteins to create multiple non-structural proteins [30]. Aside from Mpro and Ppro, SARS-CoV-2 has 3C-like cysteine protease (3CLPro), which has a 96% resemblance to SARS-CoV. These proteases are essential for viral replication and transcription, and protease inhibitors inhibiting these proteases are potential antivirals for SARS-CoV-2. The promising clinical outcomes for COVID-19 patients should be obtained by using alpha-interferon, chloroquine phosphate, arabinol, remdesivir, lopinavir/ritonavir, and anti-inflammatory drugs [31–34]. Moreover, clinical trials with these drugs should be performed on COVID-19 patients to prove their efficacy and safety as proposed for tocilizumab (**Figure 1**) [35].

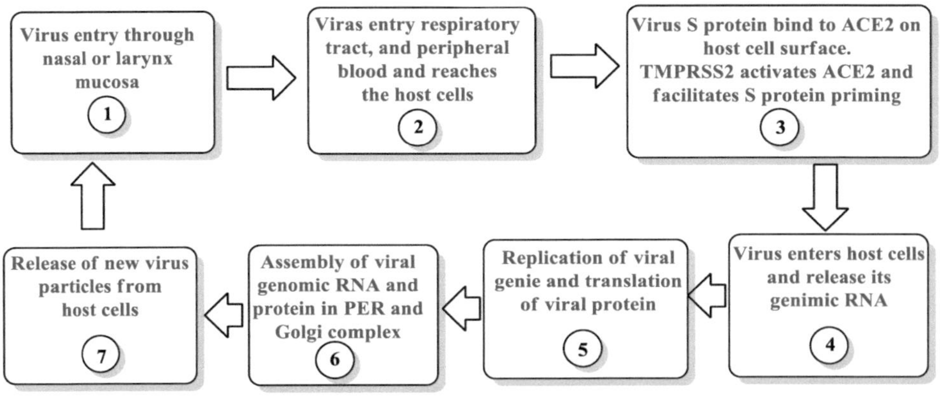

Figure 1.
Schematic diagram of the life cycle of SARS-CoV-2.

3. Transmission of SARS-CoV-2

Highest sequence similarity (~96%) was observed for the bat Coronavirus. So, it has been speculated that COVID-19 was transmitted from bats to humans. The intermediary animal host could be a pangolin or dog. COVID-19 illness is spread via intimate contact with an infected individual, as well as minute respiratory droplets emitted during coughing, sneezing, or talking [36]. Small droplets of saliva or sputum emitted from the mouth might carry large amounts of viruses that can linger in the air for lengthy periods of time and function as infection carriers. Even when a person is not in direct physical touch with the infected individual, inhaling these minute droplets causes viral infection to move from the sick to the healthy. The virus enters the human body via the eyes, nose, and mouth and spreads by encountering the virus on infected surfaces and then touching these bodily areas [37]. Environmental factors such as temperature and humidity influence viral propagation across infected surfaces [38]. The binding of homotrimer spike protein (S) on the virus's surface to ACE2 on the host's cell membrane facilitates SARS-CoV-2 entry into host cells [16]. The host cell receptor's credit is a critical predictor of the virus's tissue tropism and pathogenicity. The life cycle of SARS-CoV-2 is similar to the SARS-CoV and MERS-CoV [39]. Different strategies have been adopted to fight COVID-19.

4. Diagnosis approach and pathogenesis

COVID-19 diagnosis is a crucial step in tracking the virus and understanding its spread. This aids in the prevention of transmission as well as adequate patient care. COVID-19 is diagnosed in the first instance by observing signs and symptoms such as first loss of smell or taste or both, cough, mild to high fever, myalgia or weariness, and so on [40]. In addition, some people experience gastrointestinal problems such as vomiting, diarrhea, and nausea [41]. However, variations in the development of symptoms ranging from asymptomatic to severe instances, such as septic shock, metabolic acidosis, coagulation malfunction, and acute respiratory pneumonia-like syndrome, have been recorded often [17]. These indications and symptoms should only be used as a starting point for additional testing, not as a diagnostic tool. The recognition of symptoms in clinical conditions is the most important factor in diagnosis. Swabs are used to obtain pathological samples from the upper and lower respiratory areas (throat, oropharyngeal, nasopharyngeal, broncho-alveolar fluid, and sputum). The virus is still absent in the blood and urine of infected people, hence they are not regarded valid clinical specimens. The interlink between the temporal surge of viral load and its bio-distribution in different tissues of the body has a critical implication on the accuracy of various tests for diagnosis, according to reports of inconsistency in RTPCR test results for CoV-SARS-2 in various tissues [42] and temporal variation of test results from the same tissues [43]. SARS-spike CoV-2's surface glycoprotein binds to the ACE2 receptor and then enters the host cell. Viral particles release their DNA after entering the host cell, which is then translated into protein, and additional viral particles are created, which are then released to infect the next cells. Many assays (molecular and immunological assays) or tools have been used for the diagnosis of COVID-19 and many more are currently in development.

5. Therapeutic approaches in COVID-19

SARS-Cov-2 infections currently have no vaccinations or antiviral therapies available [44]. Because developing safe and stable vaccines takes time and the pandemic is still going on, it's critical to test and discover current medications that are already effective against SARS and MERS to determine whether they can be effectively applied to SARSCov-2. Various preclinical studies on other CoVs genetically very close to SARS-Cov-2 suggested that promising clinical outcomes for COVID-19 patients should be obtained by using several drugs including alpha-interferon, chloroquine phosphate, arabinol, remdesivir, lopinavir/ritonavir, and anti-inflammatory drugs. In a large-scale drug screening, nelfinavir has potent antiviral activity against SARS-Cov-2 [45]. Besides, praziquantel, pitavastatin, and perampanel might be effective against SARS-CoV-2. The outbreak of COVID-19 infection is related to the unavailability of specific drugs to combat this viral infection. Despite the challenges related to COVID-19 therapy, there are still several approaches being undertaken that show significant outcomes [5]. Discuss the positive impacts of some of the clinically used drugs for the COVID-19. Some drugs are in clinical trials, and some have shown significant promise in COVID-19 patients [46]. To find the solutions for COVID-19, great efforts have been made and are continued to develop vaccines, small-molecule drugs, or monoclonal antibodies that can prevent the infection [47]. In addition to drugs under clinical trials, some vaccines are expected to play a significant role in controlling the COVID-19 pandemic (**Figure 2**).

6. Remdesivir (GS-5734)

In 2009, Gilead Sciences, Inc. (USA) developed an antiviral drug called Remdesivir (RDV) to treat hepatitis B [48]. It did not indicate a desirable act against hepatitis. However, it is effective against other viruses, such as the Nipah virus, hepatitis C, and Marburg [49]. RDV is a broad-spectrum antiviral nucleoside analog, and

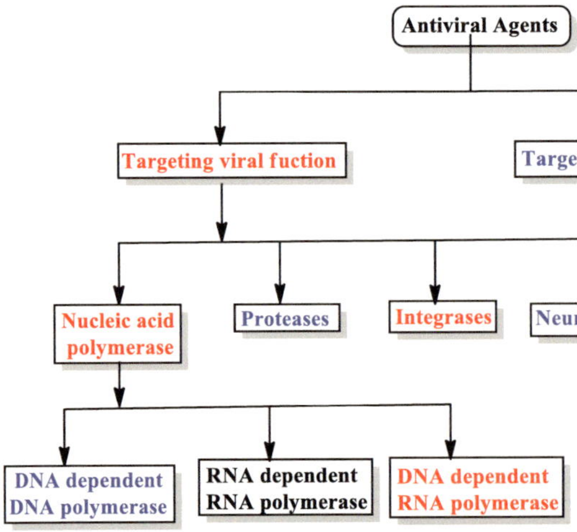

Figure 2.
Common inhibitory action of antiviral drugs.

now it is used as a treatment option for COVID-19 [50]. It is the class of polymerase inhibitors and showed activity against different RNA viruses, including SARS-CoV, MERS-CoV, Lassa fever virus, Junin virus, respiratory syncytial virus, Nipah virus, Hendra viruses, filoviruses, and Ebola viruses. RDV is a prodrug of its parent adenosine triphosphate analog, (2R,3R,4S,5R)-2-(4-aminopyrrolo(2,1-f)(1,2,4) triazin-7-yl)-3,4-dihydroxy-5-(hydroxymethyl)oxolane-2-carbonitrile (GS-441524), and has similarity to the adenine nucleic acid structurally. Both of these drugs are metabolized into the active component as nucleoside triphosphate (GS-443902) after ingestion and show antiviral activity against SARS-CoV [51]. RDV targets the viral genome replication process by acting as an RdRp inhibitor [52], RDV was used to block the RNA-dependent RNA polymerase of SARS-CoV-2. On metabolization of RDV into active nucleoside triphosphate (NTP), which competes with ATP for incorporation into nascent RNA strands, premature RNA synthesis occurs, resulting in RNA strand termination and cessation of growth [51]. RDV when tested through in vitro studies using the Vero E6 cells showed an EC_{50} value of 1.76 μM that showed its activity against SARS-CoV-2 [53]. Intravenous remdesivir treatment showed significant improvement for COVID-19. RDV and chloroquine are highly effective in the control of SARS-CoV-2 infection. In severe COVID-19 treated with RDV, improvements in the clinical finding were observed in 68% of patients [54]. However, in October 2020, the WHO removed it from the list of effective drugs in the treatment procedure of COVID-19 patients because it failed in the first trials for the treatment of COVID-19 [42]. There are still controversies regarding the results, no benefit in COVID-19 treatment using RDV; whereas, the company claims it as a promising drug for the same. After penetrating the cell, RDV as a prodrug (GS-5734) and like Favipiravir, binds to the triphosphate group under esterase, kinase, and phosphatase enzymatic reactions. These enzymes modify the structure of RDV and convert it to the active form, RDV-triphosphate (RDV-TP or GS-441524) [55]. After virus entry into the cell cytoplasm, this prodrug gets activated and loses its ability to diffuse to the intercellular space [53]. However, the primary mechanism of action of RDV against SARS-CoV-2 is unclear, and more research is necessary to understand it [56]. In an in vitro study, the combination of RDV and chloroquine (antimalarial drug) effectively inhibited SARS-CoV-2 growth in Vero E6 cells [19]. RDV is used to treat COVID-19 cases.

The combined use of RDV and IFN-β created a higher antiviral activity compared with the lopinavir/ritonavir-IFN-β combination against the MERS-CoV virus. Additionally, RDV could be better pulmonary function, cause fall lung viral loads and severe lung pathology in mice; on the contrary, lopinavir/ritonavir-IFN-β could not [57]. In two clinical studies, the use of RDV has been carried out against severe or mild respiratory infections caused by COVID-19. Recently, RDV for emergency use to treat COVID-19, including five antiviral drugs, ribavirin, RDV, sofosbuvir, galidesivir, and tenofovir, was conducted against SARS-CoV-2 RNA-dependent RNA polymerase (RdRp); these drugs showed promising results against COVID-19. Prominent adverse reactions were an acute respiratory failure, decreased glomerular filtration rate, lymphocytopenia, pyrexia, hyperglycemia, increased anemia, increased creatine, and liver transaminases. RDV given in combination with baricitinib (Janus kinase inhibitor used to hinder intracellular signaling of cytokines) was effective compared with RDV alone in terms of reducing recovery time additionally speeding improvement. RDV's parent nucleotide GS-441524 is superior and less toxic than its prodrug form and has shown efficacy [58].

7. Favipiravir

Favipiravir (Avigan or T705) is a synthetic antiviral agent that was first marketed as an anti-influenza drug in Japan. It is a derivative of pyrazine carboxamide (6-fluoro-3-hydroxy-2-pyrazine carboxamide) [59]. Due to its similarity to the purine (guanine) nucleotide, it is a type of RNA-dependent RNA-polymerase (RdRp) inhibitor. RdRp uses Favipiravir-RTP in the synthesis of mRNA strands, which can consequently stop viral protein synthesis via suppressing the translation process. Activated Favipiravir-RTP could suppress the SARS-CoV-2 RdRp enzyme and inhibit viral mRNA elongation and protein synthesis [60]. Favipiravir acts against RNA viruses by working on viral genetic copying to prevent its reproduction. A phase 3 clinical trial was involved for the treatment of COVID-19 disease using Favipiravir. For the first day, take 1800 mg twice a day, then 600 mg three times a day from the second day onward for a total of 14 days. Normalization of pyrexia, respiratory rate, and cough alleviation for at least 72 h are the key objectives [61]. The precursor of this drug known as T1105 has anti-influenza effects [62]. Drug excretion is through renal elimination and is mainly impacted by aldehyde oxidase and xanthine oxidase [62]. Favipiravir is a prodrug that is phosphorylated upon its entry into the cell and converted to an active antiviral form, favipiravir ibufuranosyl-5′-triphosphate (T-705-RTP). Favipiravir was first prescribed in Wuhan, to treat patients with SARS-CoV-2 infection. In June 2020, it was approved for mild-to-moderate COVID-19 cases in India. Favipiravir has been consumed to cure distinct viral diseases. Favipiravir was effective against some RNA viruses, such as yellow fever virus, Lisa virus, West Nile virus, Bunyavirus, arenavirus, flavivirus, filoviruses, and Ebola virus [63]. The exact mechanism of action is not clear against SARS-CoV-2. Favipiravir is considered a potential drug for COVID-19 and is currently used for COVID-19 treatment in Japan and Indonesia. Besides, its anti-influenza virus action, it stops the replication of RNA viruses such as flavi-, alpha-, filo-, bunya-, arena-, noroviruses [64]. Favipiravir showed a more powerful antiviral activity than lopinavir/ritonavir. Adverse reactions are not observed in a favipiravir therapy group. Compared with the lopinavir/ritonavir group, it had considerably fewer adverse effects. In a Japanese study, FPV was also shown to control inflammatory mediators and pneumonia progression in COVID-19 patients [65]. Severe or critical COVID-19 patients showed improvements after treating with FPV and FPV also led to improved lung histology [66].

7.1 Lopinavir/ritonavir

Lopinavir is an antiviral drug belonging to the family of protease inhibitors. It is commonly used to treat Acquired Immunodeficiency Syndrome (AIDS) and prevent HIV from spreading inside the body. Lopinavir/ritonavir (LPV/RTV) is used in combination with other antiretroviral drugs for the treatment of HIV-1 infection. In the coronavirus pandemic, when no definitive drug was proposed to treat patients, it was used in combination with Ritonavir. This LPV/RTV is branded as Kaletra. Lopinavir has a relatively short half-life in the blood and is affected by the cytochrome p450 enzyme, while Ritonavir is a protease inhibitor and reduces the Lopinavir metabolism by suppressing the function of cytochrome p450. The half-life of Lopinavir is improved, and its circulation period is increased. LPV/RTV acts as a protease inhibitor drug and inhibits the action of 3-CLpro, a chymotrypsin-like protease enzyme, that plays a vital role in the processing and interferes with the process of viral replication and its release from host cells [67–69]. LPV/RTV use is related to diverse side effects, mainly in the gastrointestinal tract. Diarrhea, impaired hepatic cell function, and pancreatitis are some of these crucial side effects.

The use of lopinavir as an emergency drug in China increased the eosinophil count among COVID-19 patients [70]. In an in silico study, LPV/RTV used as HIV protease inhibitors inhibited the main protease (MPro) of SARS-CoV-2 [71]. The LPV/RTV is being used as an emergency treatment for COVID-19 patients in some countries [72]. LPV/RTV alone or in combination with interferon (INF)-β, an inflammation regulator, has been listed by WHO as options for "solidarity" clinical trial for COVID-19. COVID-19 might benefit from LPV/RTV since it reduces viral load and improves clinical symptoms. Lung damage was also significantly reduced when LPV/RTV and umifenovir were used together [73]. A research found that while LPV/RTV therapy was associated with a better result, it did not significantly speed up the clinical progression of severe COVID-19 infection. Although the efficacy of lopinavir for COVID-19 has yet to be determined, LPV/RTV has been employed in the treatment of COVID-19 patients [57]. Now, LPV/RTV and IFN-β1b are in phase 2 for the MERS therapy. Despite the positive findings, in a recent study performed on patients with SARS-CoV-2 infection, the LPV/RTV did not provide clinical improvement compared with standard care processes [72]. Findings of LPV/RTV clinical efficacy remain limited and primarily anecdotal cases. LPV/RTV in the therapy of COVID-19 is needed as current results contradict. LPV/RTV can ameliorate the outcome of MERS-CoV infection [74]. Moreover, LPV/RTV is assumed as a therapeutic option for COVID-19 pneumonia [72]. Thus, more well-designed clinical studies are necessary to identify their efficacy as therapeutic agents for COVID-19.

7.2 Novaferon

Novaferon has potential as an antiviral drug against COVID-19. It is a synthesized protein consisting of 167 amino acids, designed on the technical basis of DNA shuffling technology. The antiviral effects of novaferon are shown alone and in combination with lopinavir/ritonavir (LPV/RTV) for COVID-19 treatment. Novaferon inhibited the viral replication in infected cells (EC_{50} = 1.02 ng/ml) and protected healthy cells from SARS-CoV-2 infection (EC_{50} = 0.1 ng/ml). Both novaferon and novaferon plus LPV/RTV groups had significantly higher SARS-CoV-2 clearance rates on day 6 than the LPV/RTV group [8].

7.3 Ribavirin

Ribavirin (Virazole) is an antiviral drug belonging to the nucleoside analogues, (1-beta-D-ribofuranosyl-1,2,4-triazole-3-carboxamide). It is a synthetic nucleoside analog with a guanosine-like structure. Ribavirin disrupts viral DNA and RNA replication, thereby inhibiting virus proliferation in the cell. Although Ribavirin's primary mechanism of action is suppressing the virus replication, and can also interfere with viral RNA capping, which depends on the presence of natural guanosine in the RNA structure. The natural guanosine in the viral RNA structure prevents the breakdown of RNA strands. Ribavirin reduces the guanosine synthesis in the cell by inhibiting the activity of the inosine monophosphate dehydrogenase enzyme, which negatively impacts virus replication [75]. Although Virazole does not entirely inhibit viral RNA synthesis, the synthesis of the viral genetic material is severely impaired. It results in significant and persistent mutations in viral RNA, which reduce the viability of the virus in host cells [76]. Besides, the presence of Ribavirin in the patient's body can reduce viral immune evasion and boost immune maintenance [77]. It is the first broad-spectrum antiviral drug against DNA and RNA viruses [75]. It is used clinically to treat HIV and hepatitis C virus (HCV) patients.

Ribavirin, which has been studied for its antiviral effectiveness against SARS-CoV-2, is used to inhibit viral RNA production and viral mRNA capping with a broad range of antiviral activity. It's a prodrug that, when metabolized, looks like purine RNA nucleotide, which prevents viral multiplication by interfering with RNA metabolism. It was discovered in a comparison study of SARS-CoV-2 patients treated with lopinavir/ritonavir (LPV/RTV) and ribavirin combination treatment [77]. Ribavirin is one of the medications used to treat COVID-19 in conjunction with either IFN alpha or LPV/RTV [46]. Using ribavirin in combination with sofosbuvir and remdesivir, docking and modeling studies revealed that ribavirin is a viable candidate medication for COVID-19 therapy [78]. Ribavirin and sofosbuvir are currently part of the therapeutic regimen to treat COVID-19 in some countries.

8. Ribavirin

Ribavirin inhibits the function of inosine monophosphate dehydrogenase, which affects the formation of guanosine triphosphate (GTP), preventing RNA and DNA viral replication. During the SARS outbreak in Hong Kong, ribavirin was utilized. With or without steroids, it was occasionally chosen. The combination of ribavirin and interferon-β, which appears to inhibit SARS-CoV replication, has shown significant efficacy in the inhibition of SARS-CoV [79]. The ribavirin triple antiviral treatment was safe and superior compared with lopinavir-ritonavir combined therapy.

9. Ribavirin

The drug showed antiviral efficacy against canine distemper virus, hepatitis C virus, Enterovirus, Chikungunya virus, and Semliki Forest virus, orthopoxvirus, influenza virus, flavi- and paramyxoviruses [80]. A study observed reduced replication of the MERS-CoV in rhesus macaques upon treatment with IFN-α2b and RBV [81]. RBV in combination with LPV/RTV was used in SARS-CoV and MERS-CoV trials [82]. In the case of SARS-CoV-2 infection, an in vitro study showed the EC_{50} of RBV as 109.50 uM [31]. A study included RBV along with LPV/RTV and IFN-α in the treatment of hospitalized COVID-19 patients. When compared with those that only received LPV-RTV, the triple treatment was found to be effective in reducing illness symptoms and viral shedding. The RBV dosage was 400 mg bid for 14 days, paired with 400 mg/100 mg of LPV/RTV + IFN-β. A research examined the effectiveness of antivirals sofosbuvir/daclatasvir and RBV in the treatment of COVID-19 patients. COVID-19 patients treated with RBV had a greater death rate (33%) than those treated with sofosbuvir/daclatasvir. A cohort study comparing RBV vs. supportive therapy stated that RBV did not help in reducing the mortality rate in COVID-19 patients [83].

10. Arbidol (Umifenovir)

It is an antiviral widely used to treat the influenza virus. Arbidol can prevent SARS-CoV-2 infection *in vitro* [10]. Lopinavir/ritonavir and Arbidol have been recommended for dealing with COVID-19 [5]. According to a research, arbidol monotherapy is more successful in treating COVID-19 than lopinavir/ritonavir. On the 14th day of therapy, no viral load was recorded in the arbidol group, compared with 44.1% viral load in patients on lopinavir/ritonavir [84]. Arbidol is used for prophylaxis and therapy of influenza and other respiratory viral infections. Arbidol and its derivative, arbidol mesylate, showed antiviral activity against SARS-CoV because they declined the reproduction of the virus in the cell cultures [85]. Arbidol was tested alone or with some antiviral agents against COVID-19, and certain positive effects were observed [5, 10]. Arbidol is a non-nucleoside fusion suppressor that interferes with cell-virus interactions [86]. The drug exerts this function by influencing the hydrogen bonds of phospholipid molecules in the cell membrane. This drug can directly impact the influenza virus. It affects the hemagglutinin (HA) protein of the influenza virus. Umifenovir, by lowering the pH threshold needed for HA to attach to the cell, prevents the conformational modifications required for the activation of this protein and causes failure in the virus entry into the cell [87, 88]. Because of the structural similarity of the SARS-CoV-2 spike proteins (SPs) to influenza HA protein, researchers speculate that Umifenovir can inhibit the binding of SARS-CoV-2 to the host cell via a similar mechanism to HA inhibition [86]. Arbidol is utilized in vitro against other viruses, such as herpes simplex virus, hepatitis C, and the Ebola virus. The suitable antiviral activity for Umifenovir against these viruses [89] tested the influence of Umifenovir, alone or combined with other agents. The effect of Arbidol on COVID-19 patients and its mechanism of action are still necessary [90]. A study reported that umifenovir monotherapy for COVID-19 patients in China resulted in negative viral conversion where the virus was not detected in 14 days [91]. Arbidol and arbidol mesylate compounds have inhibited SARS virus replication in vitro and are presently being tested in COVID-19 patients to see if they have therapeutic promise in treating pneumonia caused by SARS-CoV-2. Arbidol monotherapy was superior to LPV/RTV against COVID-19 [84]. COVID-19 patients provided with UFV along with LPV/RTV showed better outcomes compared with patients who received LPV/RTV only [46]. The UFV was not beneficial to improve the condition of the patient or viral clearance [92]. Another study suggested that arbidol + LPV/RTV were related to many adverse events. A dosage of 200 mg three times a day was considered in the majority of research. According to a meta-analysis, UFV was ineffective in lowering SARS-CoV-2 removal from infected patients in terms of diagnostic test detection and hospital duration of stay of hospitalized patients [40]. There is no evidence to support the use of UFV for improving patient-important outcomes in patients with COVID-19.

11. Darunavir

Darunavir, an anti-HIV drug, is recommended for COVID-19 treatment in Italy. It is used in a combined regimen along with cytochrome P-450 inhibitors such as ritonavir or cobicistat and confirmed their replication inhibitory effect against SARS-CoV-2. A clinical trial assessed the effectiveness of darunavir combination with other antivirals and hydroxychloroquine for COVID-19 patients. A combination of darunavir and cobicistat is also being tested [93]. PREZCOBIX®, a fixed-dose combination of darunavir and cobicistat, is also used to treat COVID-19. COVID-19 infection was recently discovered in HIV-positive individuals who were already taking darunavir, raising questions about the effectiveness of this HIV protease inhibitor. The darunavir might not be effective in preventing SARS-CoV-2 infection at the dosage of 800 mg [94].

Darunavir is a second generation of HIV-1 protease inhibitors used to prevent SARS-CoV-2 infection in vitro [17] by inhibiting viral replication at 300 μM, and this inhibition efficiency was 280-fold compared with the untreated groups. Darunavir boosted with ritonavir or cobicistat is used in HIV/AIDS treatment. The efficacy of darunavir or ritonavir is enhanced by cytochrome p450 (CYP3A) inhibition [95]. Cell experiments with darunavir showed that the drug inhibited viral replication of COVID-19 in vitro. The lopinavir/ritonavir used in the treatment of HIV/AIDS has more efficacy and tolerability than darunavir, its use in COVID-19 is limited.

11.1 Oseltamivir

Oseltamivir (Tamiflu) is an antiviral agent that is used for patients with influenza A and B. It is a protease inhibitor, which specifically inhibits the neuraminidase enzyme in the influenza virus. This enzyme has a key role in the binding of the influenza virus to the cell membrane and spread throughout the body. Therefore, Oseltamivir, by targeting neuraminidase, prevents the spread of the influenza virus and its progression inside the body [96]. This drug was used in the treatment of COVID-19 infection, which showed an appropriate effect on patients [41]. Oseltamivir has been applied in concomitant regimens with other drugs such as Hydroxychloroquine or Favipiravirs [97]. In addition to treating influenza A and B patients, this drug may also be used in severe cases. For the treatment of flu patients, Tamiflu is prescribed in a 75 mg dosage twice a day and once a day as prophylaxis. The main side effects of this drug can be nausea and headache [98]. Neuraminidase inhibitors seem beneficial for COVID-19 patients and can reduce their ventilator requirements [99]. The precise mechanism of action of Oseltamivir against COVID-19 infection is still unclear. Oseltamivir is a synthetic derivative prodrug of ethyl ester [100]. It acts as a neuraminidase inhibitor against the influenza virus and is also effective for various avian influenza virus strains [101]. An in vitro oseltamivir study on H5N1 influenza showed that the IC_{50} was 0.1–4.9 nM [102]. In vivo study involving H5N1 infection required a longer course and higher dosage of Oseltamivir. The COVID-19 originated in China during flu season, and hence earlier, many patients received oseltamivir treatment until the causative agent SARSCoV-2 was discovered. Some current clinical trials have used oseltamivir in combination with other major therapeutic drugs [31, 41].

11.2 Sofosbuvir

Sofosbuvir is an antiviral drug and RdRp inhibitor that exerts its effect by suppressing RdRp enzyme activity. A combination of Sofosbuvir with Ledipasvir is used for treating patients with genotype 1 of HCV67. Because of the similarity in the transcription and replication mechanism of the SARS-CoV-2 with HCV in host cells, physicians speculate that this drug may help treat COVID-19 patients [103]. This drug disrupts the activity of RdRp by acting like free nucleotides that are essential for viral mRNA synthesis [104]. Sofosbuvir is a potential option for COVID-19 treatment [105], and extensive clinical studies should be performed to verify the effectiveness of this drug.

12. Danoprevir

Danoprevir, an HCV N53 protease inhibitor, is authorized in China for the treatment of noncirrhotic genotype 1b chronic hepatitis C in combination with other medications. In China, only two clinical studies of danoprevir coupled with ritonavir in the treatment of SARS-CoV-2 infection were completed [8].

13. Atazanavir

In a computer simulation, atazanavir bonded more firmly to the active site of SARS-CoV-2 MPro than lopinavir, and atazanavir suppressed SARS-CoV-2 replication in a test tube. A prior trial on HIV-positive individuals found that combining atazanavir with ritonavir enhanced glucose uptake and lipid parameters while also lowering fasting glucose levels more efficiently than lopinavir-ritonavir. The atazanavir might be an alternative for lopinavir when combined with ritonavir for COVID-19 treatment. This antiviral drug is an option for COVID-19 treatment [8].

14. Baricitinib

SARS-CoV-2 penetrates host cells by receptor-mediated endocytosis, just as other viruses. AP2-related protein kinase 1 controls the process of endocytosis (AAK1). As a result, disrupting AAK1 will prevent not just viral entrance but also intracellular viral assembly. Baricitinib is a Janus kinase (JAK) inhibitor that has a high affinity for AAK1 and can inhibit it. SARS-CoV-2 infection can be treated with baricitinib, which inhibits both viral entry and the inflammatory response [106]. JAK inhibitors such as ruxolitinib and fedratinib, which are linked to baricitinib, decreased clathrin-mediated endocytosis at higher dosages, suggesting that they may not be effective at acceptable concentrations in lowering viral infectivity. Neutropenia, lymphocytopenia, and viral reactivation have all been linked to the use of baricitinib for therapeutic purposes. Because individuals infected with SARSCoV-2 had a lower absolute lymphocyte count, baricitinib may increase the risk of co-infection [107].

15. Imatinib

Blocking virus-host fusion is a promising target for the novel antiviral agents that inhibit the Abl kinase pathway [41]. In a study, imatinib, an Abl kinase inhibitor, was observed to block the replication of SARS and MERS viruses by blocking viral fusion in 2016 [108]. COVID-19 utilized the SARS-coronavirus receptor ACE2 as well as the cellular protease TMPRSS2 to get access to target cells; therefore, TMPRSS2, transmembrane serine protease 2, inhibiting medicines such imatinib might be evaluated as COVID-19 disease treatment alternatives [37].

16. Camostat mesylate

Another possible medicine that targets the fusion stage in viruses is camostat mesylate, a serine protease inhibitor. SARS-CoV-2 enters target host cells via ACE-2 receptors and/or TMPRSS2 receptors, with camostat mesylate acting as a TMPRSS2 inhibitor. It inhibits the virus's cellular entrance by downregulating the production of the SARS-CoV-2 spike (S) protein, which prevents surface fusion. SARS-CoV infection in human bronchial epithelial cells was inhibited by camostat mesylate [109]. In vitro testing revealed that camostat mesylate and E-64d (a cysteine protease inhibitor) effectively blocked SARS-CoV-2 TMPRSS2 binding. Clinical studies are now underway to compare the efficacy of hydroxychloroquine and camostat mesylate vs. hydroxychloroquine alone. Another serine protease inhibitor, nafamostat mesylate, was shown to be 15 times more effective in preventing the SARS-CoV-2 virus from infecting host cells. As a result, nafamostat mesylate can be regarded a preferable option to camostat mesylate due to its more robust antiviral activity and acceptable safety profile [37]. Disseminated

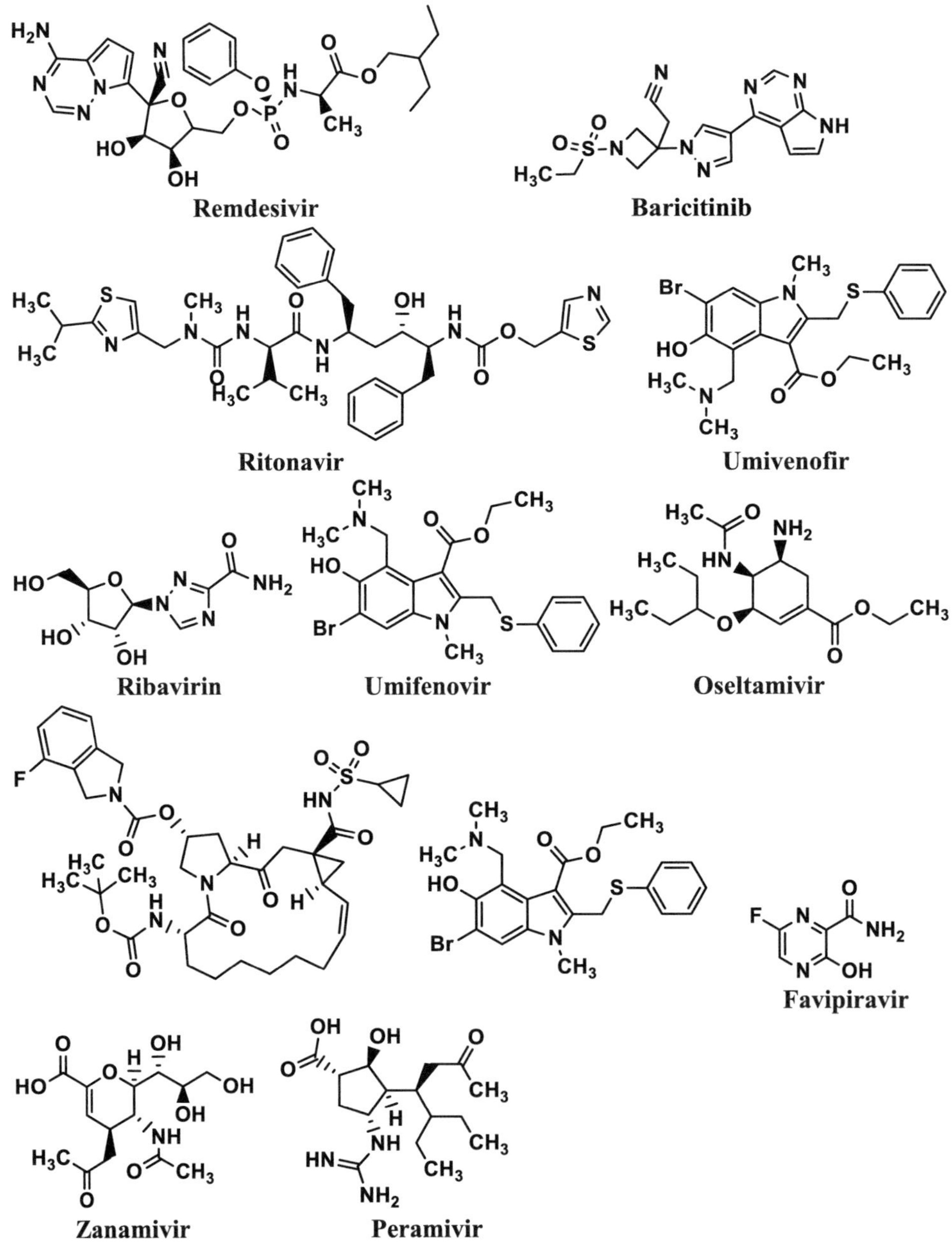

Figure 3.
Chemical structure of antiviral drugs.

intravascular coagulation is also treated with nafamostat mesylate (DIC). It will aid in the management of DIC, as seen by increased fibrinolysis in COVID-19 patients [110].

16.1 Nitazoxanide

In an in vitro research utilizing Vero E6 cells, nitazoxanide and its active component, tizoxanide, showed promise against MERS CoV and SARS CoV-2, with EC50 values of 0.92 and 2.12 μM, respectively [111]. In addition to coronaviruses, it exhibited action against norovirus, rotavirus, parainfluenza, respiratory syncytial virus, and influenza virus. This antiviral efficacy is due to the fact that the action mechanism is based on interfering with the virus's host-regulated reproduction pathways rather than the virus's particular pathways [112]. Nitazoxanide stimulates innate antiviral systems through amplification of cytoplasmic RNA sensing and type 1 IFN pathways. Nitazoxanide increases the expression of certain host systems that interfere with viral infection, allowing viruses to evade the host's cellular defenses [113]. The nitazoxanide used against influenza viruses blocks the maturation of viral hemagglutinin at the post-translational stage [112]. Even if the findings aren't promising, this medicine is used to treat some acute respiratory infections such as influenza. Although the in vitro activity of nitazoxanide against SARS-CoV-2 is promising, additional research is needed to understand its function in the management of COVID-19 (**Figure 3**).

16.2 Other antiviral drugs

Other various antiviral agents have been utilized to determine their impacts against SARS-CoV-2. Galidesivir is a nucleoside analog and a protease inhibitor [114]. This drug mechanism on COVID-19 is hypothesized to be similar to other antivirals, although its exact action mechanism is unknown. Another antiviral agent for COVID-19 is Tenofovir, which is known as an anti-influenza drug. It is an antiretroviral agent that targets DNA polymerase and inhibits virus replication [115, 116]. The action mechanism of this substance against COVID-19 requires further studies.

17. Mechanism of antivirals for SARS-CoV-2 infection

17.1 Fusion inhibitors

A fusion inhibitor is a group of antivirals that inhibit the fusion process during viral entry into the host cells. Some drugs are available with umifenovir and camostat mesylate representing antiviral activity against SARS-CoV-2 [117].

17.2 Protease inhibitors

Some protease inhibitors such as lopinavir, darunavir, and atazanavir are used against COVID-19 [118]. In a computational study, drugs such as carfilzomib, valrubicin, eravacycline, lopinavir, and elbasvir inhibited the main protease in SARS-CoV-2. Further studies are required to confirm the efficacy of these drugs. Saquinavir and other protease inhibitors such as indinavir, amprenavir, and nelfinavir might also show the same effects against COVID-19 like protease inhibitors, due to resemblance between the structures. In a computer simulation, saquinavir and indinavir were found to suppress 3CLPro activity in SARS-CoV-2 [119]. In vitro inhibition of SARS-CoV-2 was shown to be inhibited by saquinavir, indinavir, amprenavir, and nelfinavir, with nelfinavir demonstrating the greatest suppression when compared with the others. In Singapore, saquinavir has been used to treat COVID-19 patients. Two other medications, raltegravir and paritaprevir, were shown to have the ability to block 3CLPro activity in SARS-CoV-2 in a computational investigation (**Tables 1** and **2**) [120].

17.3 Reverse transcription inhibitors

Another technique for combating SARS-CoV-2 infection is to inhibit RdRp and impede viral replication by targeting the reverse transcription process. Nucleoside reverse transcriptase inhibitors (NRTIs), nucleotide reverse transcriptase inhibitors (NtRTIs), non-nucleoside reverse transcriptase inhibitors (NNRTIs), and nucleoside reverse transcriptase translocation inhibitors are a few examples of possible inhibitors (NRTTIs).

17.4 Other transcription inhibitors

Other NtRTIs with comparable structural properties to remdesivir or ribavirin, such as adefovir, tenofovir alafenamide, tenofovir disoproxil, abacavir, ganciclovir, and didanosine, exhibit antiviral effectiveness against SARS-CoV-2. NRTIs (lamivudine, stavudine, zidovudine, emtricitabine, zalcitabine, and azvudine) and NNRTIs (efavirenz, nevirapine, delavirdine, and rilpivirine) may also have antiviral activity against SARS-CoV-2 [56].

Class	Drugs	Application	Emergency use for COVID-19
Fusion inhibitor	Umifenovir (Arbidol)	Influenza	Singapore, China
Protease Inhibitor	Lopinavir	HIV	USA, Japan, Singapore, Italy, China, IPC (Lopinavir-Ritonavir fix dose)
	Darunavir	HIV-1	Italy (Darunavir-Ritonavir fix dose)
	Atazanavir	HIV-1	Singapore
	Saquinavir	HIV-1	Singapore
Nucleoside reverse transcriptase inhibitor	Emtricitabine	HIV-1	Singapore (Emtricitabine-Tenofovir fix dose)
	Azvudine	HIV-1	Singapore
Nucleotide reverse transcriptase inhibitor	Remdesivir	Ebola	WHO, IPC, USA, Singapore, Italy
	Favipiravir	(Avigan) Influenza	Singapore, Japan, Indonesia
	Ribavirin	HCV	Singapore, IPC
	Sofosbuvir	HCV	Singapore
Neuraminidase inhibitor (Virus release inhibitor)	Oseltamivir (Tamiflu)	Influenza A & B	IPC, Singapore, Indonesia

International Pulmonologists' Consensus includes the USA, India, Iran, China, Italy, Great Britain, EUA, Colombia, Egypt, Singapore, Romania, Ireland, Malaysia, Saudi Arabia, Sudan, Greece, and Bolivia.

Table 1.
Current use of existing antiviral drugs for COVID-19 [56].

Group	Drugs	Mechanism of action
Viral RNA polymerase inhibitors	Remdesivir (GS-5734)	RdRp inhibitor, prodrug, the analog of adenosine nucleotide
	Favipiravir	RdRp inhibitor, prodrug, the analog of guanosine nucleotide
Viral protein synthesis inhibitors	Ritonavir/Lopinavir	Inhibitor of protease
Inhibitors of viral entry	Hydroxychloroquine Chloroquine	Increase in endosomal pH needed for the virus/cell fusion. Interfere with cellular receptor glycosylation of SARS CoV (ACE-2)
Immunomodulators	Nitazoxanide	Interfere with host regulated pathways of virus replication, amplification of type 1 IFN pathways, and cytoplasmic RNA sensing
	Ivermectin	Inhibition of importin 1 heterodimer to inhibit the nuclear import of host and viral proteins

Table 2.
Mechanism of action of antiviral drugs used for the treatment of COVID-19.

17.5 Neuraminidase inhibitors

Oseltamivir is a neuraminidase inhibitor used in preventing influenza Neuraminidase inhibitor drugs such as oseltamivir, zanamivir, and peramivir are antiviral drugs that inhibit the viral neuraminidase enzyme and are recommended for influenza and to block the release of viral particles out of host cells. Neuraminidase inhibitors are also used as empirical treatment in MERS-CoV infection [121, 122]. However, a combination of oseltamivir with ganciclovir and lopinavir/ritonavir is used to treat COVID-19 patients [40]. A computational study also supported synergistic effects of oseltamivir-lopinavir-ritonavir combination against SARS-CoV-2 [123]. Oseltamivir is used with ceftriaxone and terbutaline to treat COVID-19 [124]. A study showed that the CT scan of the lungs of a COVID-19 patient showed significant improvement after a three-day course of oseltamivir [19]. Oseltamivir has been used either with or without antibiotics and corticosteroids against COVID-19. In a clinical trial, oseltamivir is tested with chloroquine and favipiravir [93, 125].

18. Conclusion

Nowadays, the rising SARS-CoV-2 turned into a global threat. COVID-19 targets lung cells by connecting to ACE2 protein. This protein is largely produced in some tissues such as the bile duct, liver, gastrointestinal organs, esophagus, testis, and kidney as well as lung tissue. Thus, COVID-19 may damage these organs and tissues. With the global threatening caused by COVID-19, efficient therapy against COVID-19 is quickly necessary. Nevertheless, the development of new drugs for this disease is still a huge problem for people in the world, and we have none formally approved drugs against COVID-19 now. It is very crucial to cut off the extending of this virus owing to epidemic avoidance and checking techniques. We need to develop novel drugs and to find new therapy methods to prevent this outbreak and to treat COVID-19. The extent of the current pandemic, along with other factors, such as the lack of time to develop novel and effective agents against COVID-19, the high mortality rate, possible mutations in its genetic material and severe economic shocks to societies highlight the value of testing antiviral drugs present in our drug arsenal. Some drugs that have already started with repositioning may be effective against COVId-19 as well. It is essential to address the drug-drug interaction of the drugs in COVID-19 patients with comorbidities. We hope that the continuing studies may provide solutions for the prevention and therapy against the COVID-19.

19. Future perspectives

Despite the fact that specific antiviral medications for COVID-19 have yet to be identified or authorized by the FDA, the usage of some currently existing antiviral agents that target various phases in COVID-19's life cycle might be an alternate therapeutic strategy for combating the pandemic. Fusion inhibitors, protease inhibitors, and transcription inhibitors are just a few of the interesting antiviral medication classes to investigate. Apart from antiviral medicines, various interesting techniques to treating COVID-19 are being employed, such as convalescent plasma, which has been found to reduce viral load and patient morbidity. The effects of interferon (IFN)-α/β and IL-6R inhibitor1 have also been encouraging [126–128]. The introduction of several new technologies is likely to yield good benefits. The safety of patients should be prioritized while evaluating new SARS-CoV-2 vaccinations. Nanotechnology offers an effective new route for diagnostics and treatment techniques. The more distinctive nanoparticles operate as excellent antiviral medication delivery vehicles, increasing the procedure's effectiveness. Finding appropriate diagnostic and therapeutic strategies for the fast and efficient care of severe COVID-19 patients is urgently needed [129, 130]. Different research on different CoV-induced diseases shows that using α-interferon, chloroquine phosphate, arabinol, remdesivir, lopinavir/ritonavir, and anti-inflammatory medications might result in encouraging clinical results for SARS-Cov-2 patients. Tocilizumab should be used as a therapy approach for severe COVID-19 pneumonia to achieve favorable results. Furthermore, further clinical studies with appropriate medications should be conducted on SARS-CoV-2 patients to demonstrate effectiveness and safety.

Acknowledgements

We are thankful to the Laboratory Medicine Department, Faculty of Applied Medical Sciences, Umm Al-Qura University, Makkah, 21955, Saudi Arabia, and Glocal School of Pharmacy, Glocal University, Mirzapur Pole, 247121, Saharanpur, Uttar Pradesh, India for providing necessary facilities.

Conflicts of interest

The authors declare no conflicts of interest.

Abbreviations

3CLpro	3-chymotrypsin-like protease
AAK1	AP2-associated protein kinase 1
ACE2	angiotensin-converting enzyme 2

ACEi	angiotensin-converting-enzyme inhibitors
ADR	acute respiratory distress syndrome
AIDS	acquired immunodeficiency syndrome
Cm	maximum concentration
CMV	cytomegalovirus
COVID-19	coronavirus disease 2019
DCGI	drug controller general of India
DR	drug repurposing
E	envelope protein
ER	endoplasmic reticulum
ERGIC	endoplasmic reticulum-Golgi apparatus compartment
EVD	Ebola virus disease
HA	hemagglutinin envelope glycoprotein
HAV	hepatitis A virus
HCMV	human cytomegalovirus
HCV	hepatitis-C virus
HE	hemagglutinin esterase
HSV	herpes simplex virus
ICU	intensive care unit
INF-β	interferon
Kb	kilo base pairs
M	membrane protein
MERS	Middle-East Respiratory Syndrome
Mpro	main protease
N	nucleocapsid
NNRTI	non-nucleoside reverse-transcriptase inhibitors
NRTTI	nucleoside reverse transcriptase translocation inhibitors
NtRTI	nucleotide reverse-transcriptase inhibitor
PLPro	Papain-like protease
qRT-PCR	quantitative real-time polymerase chain reaction
R0	reproductive number
RdRp	RNA-dependent RNA polymerase
RNA	ribonucleic acid
RVFV	Rift Valley fever virus
S(P)	Spike protein
S	glycoprotein spike
SARS	severe acute respiratory syndrome
SARS-CoV-2	Severe acute respiratory syndrome coronavirus 2
SPs	spike proteins
TMPRSS2	transmembrane serine protease 2
US FDA	United States Food and Drug Administration
WHO	World Health Organization

Author details

Radi Alsafi[1], Saad Alghamdi[2] and Mohammad Asif[2]*

1 Faculty of Applied Medical Sciences, Laboratory Medicine Department, Umm Al-Qura University, Makkah, Saudi Arabia

2 Glocal School of Pharmacy, Glocal University, Mirzapur Pole, Saharanpur, Uttar Pradesh, India

*Address all correspondence to: aasif321@gmail.com

References

[1] Banerjee A, Kulcsar K, Misra V, Frieman M, Mossman K. Viruses. 2019;**11**:E41

[2] Schoeman D, Fielding BC. Virology Journal. 2019;**16**:69

[3] Song Z, Xu Y, Bao L, Zhang L, Yu P, Qu Y, et al. Viruses. 2019;**11**:piiE59

[4] Nassar MS, Bakhrebah MA, Meo SA, Alsuabeyl MS, Zaher WA. European Review for Medical and Pharmacological Sciences. 2018;**22**:4956-4961

[5] Xu X, Chen P, Wang J, Feng J, Zhou H, Li X, et al. Science China. Life Sciences. 2020;**63**:457-460

[6] Wong JEL, Leo YS, Tan CC. Journal of the American Medical Association. 2020;**323**(13):1243-1244

[7] WHO. SARS-CoV-2 variants. 2020. Available from: http://www.who.int/csr/don/31-december-2020-sars-cov2-variants/en/ [Accessed: January 13, 2021]

[8] Kucukoglu K, Faydalı N, Bul D. Medicinal Chemistry Research. 2020;**29**:1935-1955

[9] Sonkar C, Kashyap D, Varshney N, Baral B, Jha HC. Clinical Medicine. 2020;**4**:1-12

[10] Dong L, Hu S, Gao J. Drug Discoveries & Therapeutics. 2020;**14**:58-60

[11] Conforti C, Giuffrida R, Dianzani C, Di Meo N, Zalaudek I. Dermatologic Therapy. 2020;**33**:1-2

[12] Zayet S, Klopfenstein T, Mercier J, Kadiane-Oussou NJ, Lan Cheong Wah L, Royer PY, et al. Infection. 2020;**49**:1-5

[13] Yesudhas D, Srivastava A, Gromiha MM. Infection. 2020;**49**:1-15

[14] Zhou P, Yang X-L, Wang X-G, Hu B, Zhang L, Zhang W, et al. Nature. 2020;**579**:270-273

[15] Hasan A, Paray BA, Hussain A, Qadir FA, Attar F, Aziz FM, et al. Journal of Biomolecular Structure & Dynamics. 2020:1-9

[16] Shereen MA, Khan S, Kazmi A, Bashir N, Siddique R. Journal of Advanced Research. 2020;**24**:91-98

[17] Chen Y, Liu Q, Guo D. Journal of Medical Virology. 2020;**92**(4):418-423

[18] Velavan TP, Meyer CG. Tropical Medicine & International Health. 2020;**25**:278-280

[19] Wu C, Liu Y, Yang Y, Zhang P, Zhong W, Wang Y, et al. Acta Pharmaceutica Sinica B. 2020;**10**:766-788

[20] Hu R, Liu C, Gong J, Cao Z. European Review for Medical and Pharmacological Sciences. 2021;**25**:2409-2414

[21] WHO. "Solidarity" Clinical Trial for COVID-19 Treatments. 2020

[22] Rossi L, Malagoli A, Biagi A, Zanni A, Sticozzi C, Comastri G, et al. Infection. 2021;**49**:287-294

[23] Chong WH, Saha BK, Ramani A, Chopra A. Infection. 2021;**49**:1-15

[24] Ghosh AK, Brindisi M, Shahabi D, Chapman ME, Mesecar AD. ChemMedChem. 2020;**15**(11):907-932

[25] Yan VC, Muller FL. ACS Medicinal Chemistry Letters. 2020;**11**:1361-1366

[26] Guo Y-R, Cao Q-D, Hong Z-S, Tan Y-Y, Chen S-D, Jin H-D, et al. Military Medical Research. 2020;7:1-10

[27] Shang J, Wan Y, Luo C, Ye G, Geng Q, Auerbach A, et al. Proceedings of the National Academy of Sciences of the United States of America. 2020;**117**:11727-11734

[28] Devaux CA, Rolain J-M, Colson P, Raoult D. International Journal of Antimicrobial Agents. 2020;**5**:105938

[29] Zhang N, Wang L, Deng X, Liang R, Su M, He C, et al. Journal of Medical Virology. 2020;**92**:408-417

[30] Hilgenfeld R. The FEBS Journal. 2014;**281**:4085-4096

[31] Wang M, Cao R, Zhang L, Yang X, Liu J, Xu M, et al. Cell Research. 2020;**30**(3):269-271

[32] Sun P, Lu X, Xu C, Sun W, Pan B. Journal of Medical Virology. 2020;**92**(6):548-551

[33] Gao J, Tian Z, Yang X. BioScience Trends. 2020;**14**(1):72-73

[34] Li G, De Clercq E. Nature Reviews. Drug Discovery. 2020;**19**:149-150

[35] Bimonte S, Crispo A, Amore A, Celentano E, Cuomo A, Cascella M. In Vivo. 2020;**34**:1597-1602

[36] Bourouiba L. JAMA. 2020;**323**:1837-1838

[37] Hoffmann M, Schroeder S, Kleine-Weber H, Müller MA, Drosten C, Pöhlmann S. Antimicrobial Agents and Chemotherapy. 2020;**64**(6): e00754-e00720

[38] Moriyama M, Hugentobler WJ, Iwasaki A. Annual Review of Virology. 2020;7:1

[39] Shamsi A, Mohammad T, Anwar S, Al Ajmi MF, Hussain A, Rehman MT, et al. Bioscience Reports. 2020;**40**:BSR20201256

[40] Huang D, Yu H, Wang T, Yang H, Yao R, Liang Z. Journal of Medical Virology. 2020;**93**(1):481-490

[41] Wang D, Hu B, Hu C, Zhu F, Liu X, Zhang J, et al. JAMA. 2020;**323**:1061-1069

[42] Wang Y, Zhang D, Du G, Du R, Zhao J, Jin Y, et al. The Lancet. 2020;**395**:1569-1578

[43] Wolfel R, Corman VM, Guggemos W, Seilmaier M, Zange S, Müller MA, et al. Nature. 2020;**581**:465-469

[44] Li JY, You Z, Wang Q, Zhou ZJ, Qiu Y, Luo R, et al. Microbes and Infection. 2020;**22**(2):80-85

[45] Li X, Geng M, Peng Y, Meng L, Lu S. Journal of Pharmaceutical Analysis. 2020;**10**:102-108

[46] Dong E, Du H, Gardner L. Lancet Infectious Diseases. 2020;**20**(5):533-534

[47] Jomah S, Asdaq SMB, Al-Yamani MJ. Journal of Infection and Public Health. 2020;**13**(9):1187-1195

[48] Badgujar KC, Ram AH, Zanznay R, Kadam H, Badgujar VC. Journal of Drug Delivery and Therapeutics. 2020;**10**:264-270

[49] Porter DP, Weidner JM, Gomba L, Bannister R, Blair C, Jordan R, et al. The Journal of Infectious Diseases. 2020;**222**:1894-1901

[50] Cao Y-C, Deng Q-X, Dai S-X. Travel Medicine and Infectious Disease. 2020;**35**:101647

[51] Amirian ES, Levy JK. One Health. 2020;**9**:100128

[52] Yin W, Mao C, Luan X, Shen DD, Shen Q, Su H, et al. Science. 2020;**368**(6498):1499-1504

[53] Saha A, Sharma AR, Bhattacharya M, Sharma G, Lee SS, Chakraborty C. Archives of Medical Research. 2020;**51**(6):585-586

[54] Grein J, Ohmagari N, Shin D. The New England Journal of Medicine. 2020;**382**:2327-2336

[55] Al-Tannak NF, Novotny L, Alhunayan A. Scientia Pharmaceutica. 2020;**88**:29-30

[56] Frediansyaha A, Tiwari R, Sharun K, Dhama K, Harapanf H. Clinical Epidemiology and Global Health. 2021;**9**:90-98

[57] Sheahan TP, Sims AC, Leist SR, Schäfer A, Won J, Brown AJ, et al. Nature Communications. 2020;**11**:220-234

[58] Yan C, Cui J, Huang L, Du B, Chen L, Xue G, et al. Clinical Microbiology and Infection. 2020;**26**(6):773-779

[59] Shiraki K, Daikoku T. Pharmacology & Therapeutics. 2020;**209**:107512

[60] Shannon A, Selisko B, Le N, Huchting J, Touret F, Piorkowski G, et al. Comm. 2020;**11**:4682-4701

[61] Arab-Zozani M, Hassanipour S, Ghoddoosi-Nejad D. BMJ Open. 2020;**10**(7):e039730

[62] Agrawal U, Raju R, Udwadia ZF. Medical Journal, Armed Forces India. 2020;**76**:370-376

[63] Furuta Y, Komeno T, Nakamura T. Proceedings of the Japan Academy, Ser. B, Physical and Biological Sciences. 2017;**93**:449-463

[64] Delang L, Abdelnabi R, Neyts J. Antiviral Research. 2018;**153**:85-94

[65] YamamuraH,MatsuuraH,NakagawaJ, Fukuoka H, Domi H, Chujoh S. Critical Care. 2020;**24**:413

[66] Takahashi H, Iwasaki Y, Watanabe T, Ichinose N, Okada Y, Oiwa A, et al. International Journal of Infectious Diseases. 2020;**100**:283-285

[67] Kumari P, Singh A, Ngasainao MR, Shakeel I, Kumar S, Lal S, et al. Clinica Chimica Acta. 2020;**510**:488-497

[68] Zhang L, Lin D, Sun X, Curth U, Drosten C, Sauerhering L, et al. Science. 2020;**368**:409-412

[69] Li H, Wang YM, Xu JY, Cao B. Zhonghua Jie He He Hu Xi Za Zhi. 2020;**43**(3):170-172

[70] Liu F, Xu A, Zhang Y, Xuan W, Yan T, Pan K, et al. International Journal of Infectious Diseases. 2020;**95**:183-191

[71] Liu X, Wang X-JJ. Genes & Genomics. 2020;**47**(2):119-121

[72] Cao X. Nature Reviews. Immunology. 2020;**20**(5):269-270

[73] Deng L, Li C, Zeng Q, Liu X, Li X, Zhang H, et al. The Journal of Infection. 2020;**9**:100128

[74] Chan JF, Yao Y, Yeung ML, Deng W, Bao L, Jia L, et al. The Journal of Infectious Diseases. 2015;**212**(12):1904-1913

[75] Graci JD, Cameron CE. Reviews in Medical Virology. 2006;**16**:37-48

[76] Crotty S, Cameron CE, Andino R. Proceedings of the National Academy of Sciences of the United States of America. 2001;**98**:6895-6900

[77] Khalili JS, Zhu H, Mak NSA, Yan Y, Zhu Y. Journal of Medical Virology. 2020;**92**:740-746

[78] Elfiky AA. Life Sciences. 2020;**248**:117477-117478

[79] Morgenstern B, Michaelis M, Baer PC, Doerr HW, Cinatl J Jr. Biochemical and Biophysical Research Communications. 2005;**326**:905-908

[80] Galli A, Mens H, Gottwein JM, Gerstoft J, Bukh J. Scientific Reports. 2018;**8**:1-13

[81] Falzarano D, de Wit E, Rasmussen AL, Feldmann F, Okumura A, Scott DP, et al. Nature Medicine. 2013;**19**:1313-1317

[82] Yao T, Qian J, Zhu W, Wang Y, Wang G. Journal of Medical Virology. 2020;**92**:556-563

[83] Tong S, Su Y, Yu Y, Wu C, Chen J, Wang S, et al. International Journal of Antimicrobial Agents. 2020;**56**:106114

[84] Zhu Z, Lu Z, Xu T, Chen C, Yang G, Zha T, et al. The Journal of Infection. 2020;**81**:e21-e23

[85] Khamitov RA, La Loginova S, Shchukina VN, Borisevich SV, Maksimov VA, Shuster AM. Voprosy Virusologii. 2008;**53**:9-13

[86] Vankadari N. International Journal of Antimicrobial Agents. 2020;**56**:105998-105998

[87] Boriskin Y, Leneva I, Pecheur EI, Polyak S. Current Medicinal Chemistry. 2008;**15**:997-1005

[88] Leneva IA, Russell RJ, Boriskin YS, Hay AJ. Antiviral Research. 2009;**81**:132-140

[89] Pécheur E-I, Borisevich V, Halfmann P, Morrey JD, Smee DF, Prichard M, et al. Journal of Virology. 2016;**90**:3086-3092

[90] Costanzo M, De Giglio MA, Roviello GN. Current Medicinal Chemistry. 2020;**27**:4536-4541

[91] Kadam RU, Wilson IA. Proceedings of the National Academy of Sciences of the United States of America. 2017;**114**:206-214

[92] Lian N, Xie H, Lin S, Huang J, Zhao J, Lin Q. Clinical Microbiology and Infection. 2020;**26**:917-921

[93] Lu H. BioScience Trends. 2020;**14**(1):69-71

[94] Riva A, Conti F, Bernacchia D, Pezzati L, Sollima S, Merli S, et al. Pharmacological Research. 2020;**157**: 104826

[95] Santos JR, Curran A, Navarro-Mercade J, Ampuero MF, Pelaez P, Pérez-Alvarez N, et al. AIDS Research and Human Retroviruses. 2019;**35**:513-518

[96] Whitley RJ, Hayden FG, Reisinger KS, Young N, Dutkowski R, Ipe D, et al. The Pediatric Infectious Disease Journal. 2001;**20**:127-133

[97] Rosa SGV, Santos WC. Revista Panamericana de Salud Pública. 2020;**44**:1-7

[98] Srinivas P, Sacha G, Koval C. Cleveland Clinic Journal of Medicine. 2020;**88**:1-5

[99] Pagliano P, Sellitto C, Conti V, Ascione T, Esposito S. Infection. 2021;**49**:1-10

[100] Schade D, Kotthaus J, Riebling L, Kotthaus J, Müller-Fielitz H, Raasch W, et al. Journal of Medicinal Chemistry. 2014;**57**:759-769

[101] Ward P, Small I, Smith J, Suter P, Dutkowski R. The Journal of Antimicrobial Chemotherapy. 2020;**55**:i5-i21

[102] Govorkova EA, Ilyushina NA, McClaren JL, Naipospos TSP, DouangngeunB,WebsterRG.Antimicrobial Agents and Chemotherapy. 2009;**53**:3088-3096

[103] Nourian A, Khalili H. Acta BioMedica Atenei Parmensis. 2020;**91**:239-240

[104] Zuccaro V, Lombardi A, Asperges E, Sacchi P, Bruno R. Expert Opinion on Drug Metabolism & Toxicology. 2020;**16**:97-101

[105] Roozbeh F, Saeedi M, Alizadeh-NavaeiR,Hedayatizadeh-OmranA, Merat S, Wentzel H, et al. The Journal of Antimicrobial Chemotherapy. 2021;**76**:753-757

[106] Richardson P, Griffin I, Tucker C, Smith D, Oechsle O, Phelan A, et al. Lancet. 2020;**395**:e30

[107] Praveen D, Chowdary PR, Aanandhi MV. International Journal of Antimicrobial Agents. 2020;**55**(5):105967

[108] Coleman CM, Sisk JM, Mingo RM, Nelson EA, White JM, Frieman MB. Journal of Virology. 2016;**90**:8924-8933

[109] Kawase M, Shirato K, van der Hoek L, Taguchi F, Matsuyama S. Journal of Virology. 2012;**86**:6537-6545

[110] Asakura H, Ogawa HJ. Thrombosis and Haemostasis. 2020;**18**(6):1521-1522

[111] Yavuz S, Unal S. Turkish Journal of Medical Sciences. 2020;**50**:611-619

[112] Rossignol J-F. Journal of Infection and Public Health. 2016;**9**:227-230

[113] Jasenosky LD, Cadena C, Mire CE, Borisevich V, Haridas V, Ranjbar S, et al. iScience. 2019;**19**:1279-1290

[114] Zumla A, Chan JF, Azhar EI, Hui DS, Yuen K-Y. Nature Reviews. Drug Discovery. 2016;**15**:327-347

[115] Drosu NC, Edelman ER, Housman DE. Proceedings of the National Academy of Sciences of the United States of America. 2020;**117**:12368-12374

[116] Clososki GC, Soldi RA, Silva RMD, Guaratini T, Lopes JN, Pereira PR, et al. Journal of the Brazilian Chemical Society. 2020;**31**:1552-1556

[117] Zhang L, Liu Y. Journal of Medical Virology. 2020;**92**:479-490

[118] Harrison C. Nature Biotechnology. 2020;**38**:379-381

[119] Hall DC Jr, Ji HF. Travel Medicine and Infectious Disease. 2020;**35**:101646

[120] Ko WC, Rolain JM, Lee NY, Chen P-L, Huang C-T, Lee PI, et al. International Journal of Antimicrobial Agents. 2020;**55**:105933

[121] Bleibtreu A, Jaureguiberry S, Houhou N, Boutolleau D, Guillot H, Vallois D, et al. BMC Infectious Diseases. 2018;**18**:331

[122] Chow EJ, Doyle JD, Uyeki TM. Critical Care. 2019;**23**:214

[123] Muralidharan N, Sakthivel R, Velmurugan D, Gromiha MM. Journal

of Biomolecular Structure & Dynamics. 2021;**39**:2673-2678

[124] Mousavi SH, Shah J, Giang HT, Al-Ahdal TMA, Zahid SU, Temory F, et al. Lancet Infectious Diseases. 2020;**20**(6):657-658

[125] Mitjà O, Clotet B. The Lancet Global Health. 2020;**8**(5):e639-e640

[126] Casadevall A, Pirofski L-A. The Journal of Clinical Investigation. 2020;**130**(4):1545-1548

[127] Indari O, Jakhmola S, Manivannan E, Jha HC. Frontiers in Pharmacology. 2021;**12**:632677

[128] Jakhmola S, Indari O, Chatterjee S, Jha HC. SN Comprehensive Clinical Medicine. 2020;**2**(11):2137-2146

[129] Jones BM, Ma ESK, Peiris JSM, Wong PC, Ho JCM, Lam B, et al. Clinical and Experimental Immunology. 2004;**135**:467-473

[130] Xia S, Liu M, Wang C, Xu W, Lan Q, Feng S, et al. Cell Research. 2020;**30**:343-355

Chapter 4

Immunoinformatics and Computer-Aided Drug Design as New Approaches against Emerging and Re-Emerging Infectious Diseases

Mohammed Othman Aljahdali,
Mohammad Habibur Rahman Molla and Foysal Ahammad

Abstract

Infectious diseases are initiated by small pathogenic living germs that are transferred from person to person by direct or indirect contact. Recently, different newly emerging and reemerging infectious viral diseases have become greater threats to human health and global stability. Investigators can anticipate epidemics through the advent of numerous mathematical tools that can predict specific pathogens and identify potential targets for vaccine and drug design and will help to fight against these challenges. Currently, computational approaches that include mathematical and essential tools have unfolded the way for a better understanding of newly originated emerging and re-emerging infectious disease, pathogenesis, diagnosis, and treatment option of specific diseases more easily, where immunoinformatics plays a crucial role in the discovery of novel peptides and vaccine candidates against the different viruses within a short time. Computational approaches include immunoinformatics, and computer-aided drug design (CADD)-based model trained biomolecules that offered reasonable and quick implementation approaches for the modern discovery of effective viral therapies. The essence of this review is to give insight into the multiple approaches not only for the detection of infectious diseases but also profound how people can pick appropriate models for the detection of viral therapeutics through computational approaches.

Keywords: immunoinformatic, pharmacophore modeling, molecular docking, quantum mechanism, peptide and vaccine design

1. Introduction

Infectious diseases are types of transmissible or communicable diseases mainly caused by pathogenic living microorganisms. The disease not only can transmit from animal to animal but also transfer from animal to human through the parasite, virus, and bacteria [1]. The sudden invasion of infectious disease is a critical objective for the quietly alive of people in the ground [2]. However, it is not always an easy task to identify and anticipate the small pathogenic like small particles that are responsible for sudden chronic situations increasing incidence in geographic range [3]. Therefore, the situation demands to identify the unpredictable appearance of new infectious diseases as soon as possible that can utilize for further development of new therapeutic agents. Before identifying the causal infectious agents, the inevitable, but unpredictable, the appearance of newly emerging and re-emerging infectious diseases should be understood. The term emerging infectious diseases (EID) refers to infections that are newly arrived or evolved in a certain population, whose incidence can rapidly increase worldwide and threaten for future. On the other hand, infectious diseases that were previously appeared in the population and gradually decrease the incident but currently expanding into new geographical, host, or vector immensely that called re-emerging viral disease [4]. The virus disease has been recognized mostly from zoonotic by infecting a human. The primary source of zoonotic virus from farm and wild animal causes disease in human. Approximately 60 to 75% of known human pathogens ascend from animals [5]. Animal reservoirs have been involved in numerous virus families such as Filoviridae, Arenaviridae, Flaviviridae, and Bunyaviridae that were responsible to transmitted virus animals to humans *vice versa*. Most of the viruses abovementioned can be occurred emerging or re-emerging diseases, which do not have any specific therapeutic agents. Therefore, the development of vaccines and antimicrobial drugs candidates is an urgent issue that can control or prevent emerging or re-emerging diseases as soon as possible.

With the advancement of computational biology and immunoinformatics, rapid detection of pathogens and related proteins responsible for the disease has been developed. The technology helps to determine pathogen types within a short time and is utilized for therapeutic development. For example, immunoinformatic approaches can predict epitopes and their target protein is the recent advancement in vaccine design and development process that controlled the uses of antigen variation as well as hitting conserved epitopes [6]. It mainly designs immunogens by the protective responses of the target-specific receptor [7]. In the consequences of DNA virus infection and replication, it first attaches to the outer cell of the host through the protein receptor and replicates DNA by using host cell enzymes [8]. Finally, DNA goes to messenger RNA and translates it into a viral protein. Complete viral particles have converted by the replicate DNA and viral protein when new viruses were released from the host cell [9]. Additionally, RNA viruses are operated precisely as messenger RNA to make viral proteins. This mechanism of viral infections can be predicted through computational tools and immunoinformatics can identify desired epitopes for designing vaccines against the infections. On the other hand, computer-aided drug design (CADD) consists of a computer-assisted *de novo* design that can predict several models based on drug-target interaction network and help to early stage of drug design through molecular docking, similarity search methods, and deep learning-based model. The confirmation of ligand and the target protein can be initially predicted through molecular docking [10]. However, the performance of docking is quietly dependent on various types of receptors as well as acting best for the hydrophobic vs. hydrophilic pockets, which can also be determined by the CADD approaches.

Furthermore, consistent advancement of medical and pharmaceutical research has been playing an important role in the proper solution of several diseases but remained some problems with viral disease that may suffer or burden to public and animal health [11]. Therefore, computational techniques have opened a new avenue for minimizing the problems of drug discovery. The pharmaceutical industry has been starting to take up help from computational methods for drug design and development, drug repurposing, enlightening medicinal efficiency, and clinical trial [12]. The increasing data digitalization in a pharmaceutical company can be solved clinical problems that can also be done through computational methods. They have maintained a large volume of data for solving infectious diseases by their automation. The extremely widespread diseases remain virus diseases that cause infection by a type of microorganisms [13]. The most prominent type of virus diseases is common cold, while another one is an infection of virus that affected the upper respiratory tract such as nose and throat [14]. Furthermore, antibiotics have a magical role in preventing bacterial disease and infections but have no effects on viral disease. The most significant challenge to the researcher is finding out the epidemiology, vaccine design, and eradication in a worthwhile manner [15].

2. Infectious disease

Infectious disease is a kind of disorder that is caused by one or more organisms. Many organisms consist of our body where some are normally helpful or infectious with parasites and viruses as well as bacteria and fungi [16]. SARS, recently emerged SARS-CoV-2, tuberculosis (TB), HIV/AIDS, influenza, Chickenpox, the common cold, and Hepatitis A and B are some examples of infectious diseases that can easily transmit from human to human or animal to human under adverse conditions and help to cause diseases. However, the animals or insects are directly or indirectly responsible for transmission to these organisms. Contaminated food items have exposed some infectious to the new environment and move apart from diseases [17]. There are various signs and symptoms of infectious diseases such as fever, fatigue, coughing, muscle aches, and diarrhea, and so on. Infectious diseases can be remedied or controlled by vaccines, but it takes a long time for application. Most infectious diseases controlled by consciousness of diseases such as handwashing can help to protect from many infectious diseases [18].

2.1 Global burden of infectious diseases

Over the last few centuries, millions of people have lost their lives to infectious diseases throughout the world. The risk of public health has been reduced and controlled through the improvement of the sanitation system, the progress of antibiotics and vaccines, living condition, and food quality, which is linked to the socioeconomic modernization of these societies [16]. Despite the improvement of health care facilities and surveillance systems, there have been some uncertainties that still now lead to an increase the human mortality from infectious diseases. The current threat to global human health is zoonoses [19]. The mutually transmitted 200 diseases occurred between humans and animals. The zoonotic disease has been increasing due to the overpopulation, wars, and food scarcity that are associated with humans who contract face to face [20]. However, the global death increased in 2010 due to infectious disease from HIV/AIDS that constitutes 1.5 million, and hereby malaria raised to 1.17 million [21]. At the same time, about 152,000 people died by the neglected tropical disease, and 1.2 million people died of tuberculosis [22]. Long-term illness, disability, and social stigma are occurring from poverty and are renamed by infectious diseases of poverty (IDoP). Moreover, coronavirus disease 2019 (COVID-19) has the main worldwide burden in this era expressing itself as a pandemic and killed almost 4,825,433 people from the beginning and has been infecting till now [23]. The global health system has been affected by the pandemic due to the unintentional interruption of service delivery. Until now, a total of 369 infectious diseases have been identified based-on mortality and the estimation of life expectancy according to global burden diseases in 2020. There are several factors responsible for diseases that have compiled during the COVID-19 pandemic by analyzing 286 causes of death, about 369 injuries and infections, and 87 threat issues from the 204 nations [24].

2.2 Emerging and re-emerging infectious disease

Several infectious pathogens have been halting their activities from the initial discovery and reappearance after a long and short period in several places [25]. Among them are Emerging and Re-Emerging Infectious Diseases (EIDs). They are types of infections that have newly originated or previously existed in a population that is rapidly increasing in incidence or geographic range. The newly emerging and re-emerging viral disease has threatened public and animal health, which is increasing due to human activities [26]. There are many associated factors related to the spread of infectious viral disease from one place to another place such as population migration, urbanization, public gathering, poverty, malnutrition, increased domestic and global connectivity and environmental changes, and so on [4]. The alteration of genetic phenomena has also been responsible for to spread of disease to a greater extent. Most of the infectious diseases have been estimated in zoonotic that constituted 60 to 70% of total diseases [27]. Hence, the animal virus also mutated with a human virus that accelerates infectious viral disease and generates the chronic problem. As a result, thousands of people die without medicine or even without knowing about the threat [28]. Novel pathogens have occurred due to unplanned urbanization of habitat destruction that enhances the contact or susceptibility to infections between human and animal vectors of viral diseases herewith the lack of immunity of these communities [29]. However, many pathogens re-emerging again after many years such as Chikungunya and Zika virus.

2.3 History of emerging and re-emerging virus

Initially, there was an outbreak of chikungunya between 1963 and 1973 with serious arboviral illness and it re-emerged in 2006, which firstly was observed in the East African strain of chikungunya [30]. Similarly, the Zika virus was initially associated with a serious illness that has conducted by serological studies in 1960 and after a long time, it has identified and reported from Brazil in 2015 [31]. The discovery of novel pathogens in the world has not been clogged and they are associated with economic cost reflect the burden for many developed and underdeveloped countries (**Table 1**). The high cost of medical and intensive care has been banned for all kinds of work from the affected region.

2.4 Factor influences emerging and re-emerging viral bond diseases

Viral diseases have chorionic effects on public health worldwide. The annual death has been attributed to about 20 million by infectious diseases [34]. Most of the death

Family	Pandemic Year	Viruses	Probable/mode of transmission	Outbreak potential
Bunyaviridae	1917	Ganjam virus or Nairobi sheep disease virus (NSDV)	Tick-borne	Yes*
	1954	Bhanja virus	Tick-borne	Yes*
	2009	SFTS virus	Tick-borne	Yes
	1719	Chobar Gorge virus	Tick-borne	No
	2008	EEV	Arthropod-borne	No
	2004	Cat Que. virus	Arthropod-borne	Yes*
	1957	Kaisodi virus	Tick-borne	Yes*
	1955	Umbre virus	Arthropod-borne	Yes*
	1965	Ingwavuma virus	Arthropod-borne	No
	1957	Chittoor virus	Tick-borne	Yes*
	1964	Thottapalayam virus	Rodent-borne	No
Nairoviridae	1944	CCHFs virus	Tick-borne, human to human	Yes
Flaviviridae	1955	Yellow fever	Arthropod-borne	Yes
	1947	Zika virus	Arthropod-borne, mother to child, sexual route	Yes
	1957	KFD	Tick-borne	Yes
	1952	JE	Arthropod-borne	Yes
	1992	Dengue	Arthropod-borne	Yes
	1966	Bagaza virus	Arthropod-borne	Yes*
Paramyxoviridae	1968	Influenza - (H3N2) v alias	Air-borne	Yes
	2004	Avian Influenza	Air-borne	Yes
	2006	Influenza -Avian (H5N1)	Air-borne	
	1956	RSV	Air-borne	Yes
	1953	Quaranfil virus	Tick-borne	Yes*
	late 1950s	Parainfluenza 1–4	Air-borne	Yes*
	2009	Influenza H1N1	Air-borne	
	1962	Enterovirus-D68	Air-borne	Yes
Paramyxoviridae	2001	Nipah virus	Human to human	Yes
			Direct contact/consumption of infected bat/fruit infected with bat	
Picornaviridae	1953	Human rhinovirus A, B and C	Air-borne	Yes
	1957	Hand, foot and mouth disease	Direct contact, feco-oral route	Yes
	1948–49	Coxsackie-A21 virus	Feco-oral route	Yes
	1948–1949	Coxsackie-A10 virus	Feco-oral route	Yes
	1977	Sapoviruses	Feco-oral route	Yes
	1973	Rota	Feco-oral route	Yes
	1997	Polio and non-polio flaccid paralysis	Feco-oral route	Yes

Family	Pandemic Year	Viruses	Probable/mode of transmission	Outbreak potential
Caliciviridae	1936	Noroviruses	Feco-oral route	Yes
Hepadnaviridae	2007	Hepatitis KIs virus new and vaccine escape mutants of HBV	Blood-borne	Yes
Togaviridae	1740	Rubella virus	Air-borne	Yes
	2005	Chikungunya virus	Arthropod-borne	Yes
Poxviridae	1934	Buffalopox virus (orthopoxvirus)	Direct contact	Yes
	1958	Human monkey pox	Air-borne	
Parvoviridae	1975	Human parvovirus 4	Parenteral transmission?	Yes
Arenaviridae	1934	LCMV	Rodent-borne	Yes*
Herpesviridae	1934	CMV	Direct contact	Yes
	1974	Chickenpox (varicella) VZV	Air-borne, direct contact	Yes
Rhabdoviridae	1965	Chandipura virus	Arthropod-borne	Yes
Reoviridae	1963	Kammavanpettai virus (orbiviruses)	Tick-borne	No
Coronaviridae	2003	SARS Coronavirus	Air-borne	Yes
	2019	Coronavirus disease-2019 (COVID-19)	Air-borne	Yes
Polyomaviridae	1953	Polyoma-like virus	Human to human	Yes
Phenuiviridae	1931	Rift valley fever	Blood-borne	Yes

Table 1.
Emerging and re-emerging virus figure out with the inauguration periods [32, 33].

not only occurred by acute respiratory tract infection and gastrointestinal infections but also come out through tuberculosis and malaria that remained unchanged till now [35]. Many factors have been leading to emerging and re-emerging infectious diseases such as demographic factors, population distribution, sexual behavior, childcare, food-borne and water-borne diseases, ecological alteration and land use, chronic manifestations, enhanced pathogen detection, microbial evolution, and failure of community health scheme and bioterrorism shown in **Figure 1** [36]. The variations of the global population have been contributing to the growth and density in per capita, resettlement to the city area, international tourism, migration, and retaining density that directly or indirectly leads to the infectious virus disease [37]. However, there are some intentional reasons too responsible for the emerging and re-emerging virus such as the deliverance of sexual practice, enhanced childcare beyond the family, alcohol and drug abuse, food supply, transportation, and immunization practices [32]. Moreover, the environmental and land use causes of global warming, deforestation, and natural disasters such as floods, drought, and *El Nino* effect will be the lead to current and future infectious diseases [38]. The invention of modern technology can manifest the infectious diseases that are prolonging the life of people in the world. The use of new molecular techniques has enhanced to detection of fastidious and uncultivatable organisms [39]. As a result, a variety of pathogens were discovered in a short time. Nowadays, microbiomes naturally adapt to their environment for survival causing a wide range of microorganisms that

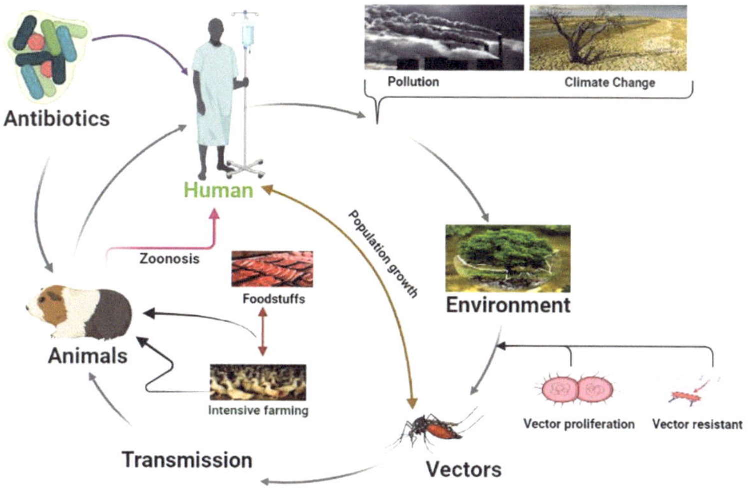

Figure 1.
Representing different factors that influence the activities of emerging and re-emerging viral bond diseases.

have become resistant to diseases [40]. Consequently, it can alter the present situation and convey the hazardous situation for human life.

2.5 Preventive measures of emerging and re-emerging disease

Due to the degradation of the environment, many contagious infections spread out the world for a long time. However, some diseases have been treated through the antibiotic and controlled with the vaccine but most of the disease's remedies remained unchanged still now [41]. Scientists and researchers have been searching for a new link in an infectious chain through their internal activities. The consumption of raw food is one of the triggers of infectious diseases. Raw food usually has lots of harmful microorganisms that can hamper your normal life within a short time [41]. Several factors have been contributing to the vast range of emerging and non-emerging diseases such as changes in human behaviors, enhancement of technology, change in the land pattern and economic progress, tourism, microbial change, and collapse of public health measures [41]. However, the prevention and control have been taken by the Pan American Health Organization (PAHO) that regulates some measures of emerging and re-emerging diseases [42]. First, there is need to increase and strengthen regional surveillance networks that control infectious diseases from one place to another place. Later, the rapid responses of infectious diseases thereby enhance the laboratory equipment and training. Moreover, the development of applied research fields can prevent the disease through the rapid diagnosis of epidemiology as well as prevention [43]. Finally, the enhancement of regional capacity and strength can control and prevent emerging and re-emerging diseases through effective implementation [44].

2.6 Traditional methods of preventing emerging and re-emerging disease

Emerging viral diseases have occurred previously and resultant pandemics where plant derived was the first choice for treatment. Around 1500 BC, Egyptians were started herbal drug preparation by the medicinal plant where later Greek and Roman have improved it [45]. Emerging infectious diseases have been treated traditionally by the medicinal plant before inventing a drug or vaccine [46, 47]. In China, it was widely used to deal with infectious diseases. They believe that it boosts the immune system and protects the virus to enter the respiratory tract [48]. Many medicinal herbs have a unique antiviral effect and are used as a substitute for an antimicrobial drug against infectious diseases. They have used the whole body of herb or part of the plant such as leaves, roots, bark, fruit, seeds, flowers, and so on, for preventing and healing respiratory tract infections [49]. In the modern time, it has been perceived that the traditional drug safer and healthier than synthetic drug those comes from plant-based traditional medicine. Plant-derived drug discovery has been renowned for the last decade [50]. It is considered that plant products will be an indispensable source of a new drug in the future.

3. Computer-aided drug design approaches

3.1 Pharmacophore modeling

Pharmacophore is one of the most promising *in silico* concepts, which is utilized to screen large compound libraries. The process includes combining medicinal chemistry and computational chemistry that can screen and optimize lead compounds for the development of the final drug candidate [50]. The pharmacophore model can function in two ways such as ligand-based modeling and structure-based modeling (**Figure 2**). The ligand-based model is fully based on computerized for simplifying drug discovery in the macromolecular target structure [51]. It generates three-dimensional (3D) structures for interacting ligand and macromolecules. Software such as Schrödinger (https://www.schrodinger.com/) and so on are used for pharmacophore drug design. Furthermore, the direct interaction of 3D structure with macromolecule ligand complex is arranged by structure-based pharmacophore modeling. The investigation of the complementary chemical feature of the active site and their spatial relationships and assembly with the selected feature will be generated using the structure-based pharmacophore modeling [52]. Discovery studio is usually practiced for the implementation of the structure-based pharmacophore method. The catalyst feature of pharmacophoric is H-bond acceptor, H-bond donor, and hydrophobic. Virtual-based pharmacophore screening has been reducing the possibility of arising problems about inadequate consideration of protein selectivity with the optimizing

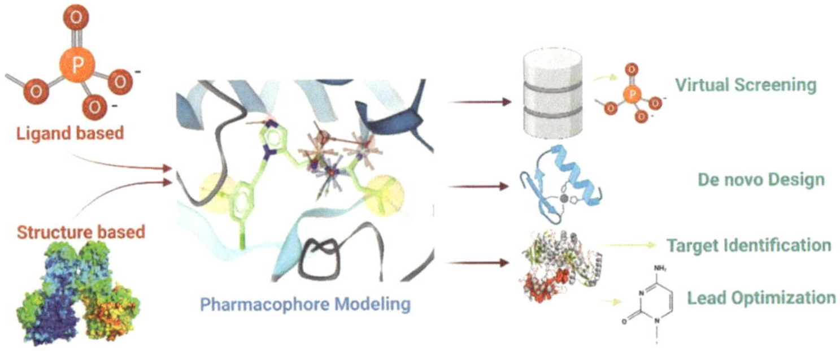

Figure 2.
Pharmacophore model-based virtual screening process for identification of small molecular candidates against a specific disease.

score and insufficient design by leading a tolerance radius for each feature [53]. The main purpose of pharmacophore model-based virtual screening is to count the highest molecules hit, which has similar or nearest the target.

3.2 Virtual screening

3.2.1 Molecular docking

In modern drug design and discovery, molecular docking is one of the foremost strategies to find the best molecules for a specific target. It assists to predict the interaction of protein and a ligand at the bond stage. Molecular docking is used to calculate the scoring function by sampling algorithms shown in **Figure 3** [54]. Furthermore, it is reasonable, time demanding, and effective more than any conventional technology. The computer-based drug designing method predicts the function of any individual protein of interest that conducts a very comprehensive approach [55]. It has various applications among them protein-ligand docking is one of them. It is primarily designed to predict the binding of small drug molecules from medicinal herbs or plants, invertebrates, and so on to target proteins [56]. The number of diseases is caused by the harmful receptors; hence, docking is designed to inhibit or induce the target protein. However, the discovery of drugs in the traditional way is very expensive because of the need to search a large volume of compounds to select against a particular protein for the proper binding interaction and targeting diseases [57]. Therefore, computerized docking can screen virtually thousands of compounds in a short time by experimental high-throughput screening and confirmed the ligand and receptor for stable binding. It also provides the knowledge-based scoring functions that interact with atom pairs between protein and ligand complexes along with three-dimensional structure. There are several purposes of molecular drug design [58]. Among them, three are main purposes such as predicting the active ligand, binding affinities, and identifying new ligand. Based on molecular

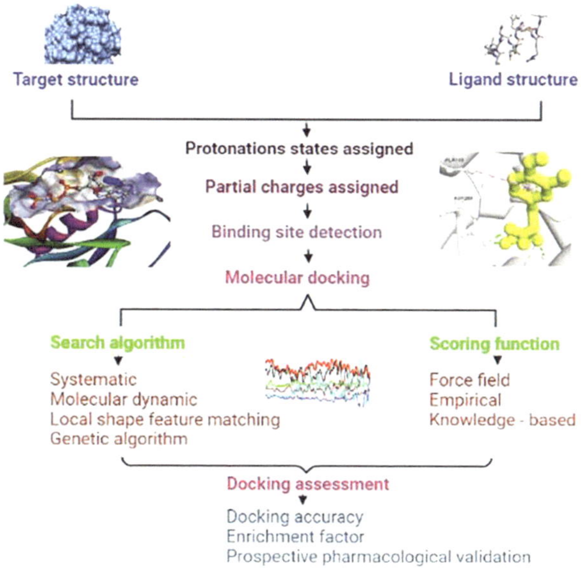

Figure 3.
Molecular docking-based screening approaches of small molecules against a specific target.

docking, it has numerous applications such as documenting the lowest free energy structure for the receptor-ligand complex, estimating the differential binding of a ligand of two separate macromolecular receptors, the geometry of the specific ligand-receptor complex, lead generation and optimization for future drug candidate, and so on [59].

3.2.2 Molecular dynamic simulation

Molecular dynamics (MD) simulation is a computer-based simulation technique that mainly analyzed the physical motion of atoms and molecules across a specific conformational space [60]. MD simulation is the unique way to drug discovery in the present era that led to work in a wet lab after computer simulation. The MD simulation ensures the detail of the dynamic properties of selected protein and plays a key role in the modeling and characterization of a protein [61]. The MD simulation also helps to determine the stability of a ligand to the active site of the targeted macromolecules. Moreover, MD simulation not only provides the information of the ligand optimization process at the qualitative level but also estimates accurately in ligand binding affinities. The tiny, microscopic event (protein-ligand interaction and molecular motion) occurs with a micro- or nano-second time scale that is not possible to determine without the technique [62]. Finally, dynamic simulation is a faster, reasonable, widely accessible, and perfect method for drug design *in silico* techniques. Moreover, it provides information of atomic position with respect to time. It usually explains the atomic and molecular properties of the protein, drug-target interaction, solvation of compound, and conformational changes that a receptor expresses in various conditions [63]. It works on the base of Newtonian mechanics (NM), which is related to the motion of large particles. The force fields are an important factor for MD simulation, which are mainly a set of the potential energy function for employing the relation between structure and potential energy. The particles are coordinated by the system of mathematical expression [64]. The computerized technique (force and energy) is used for building blocks that combined bonded and non-bonded interaction. Force acting on each atom was counted by using the force field of molecular machines that were developed through the four principal such as Born-Oppenheimer method, bond length, and bond angle, and potential energy of the surface molecule and atom type [65].

3.2.3 Quantum mechanics

Quantum mechanics has been leading a valuable method for drug discovery through characterizing the structure, dynamics, and energies of protein-ligand interaction [66]. In the medicinal industry and academic research, it is an inevitable part of drug design that fixes the problem by calculating chemical reactivity and helps to optimize structure [67]. The new drug candidate has been chosen by molecular mechanics (MM) but the quantum mechanics (QM)-based approach provides accurate accuracy and efficiency in the complexity of protein-ligand interactions [68]. Furthermore, it does not provide only the estimation of being affinities, determining ligand energies and bioactive conformations, refinement of molecular geometries but also added scoring docked ligand poses, describing molecular similarity, structure-activity, relationship analysis, and ADMET prediction in the activities of drug design [69]. QM is getting popular day by day in drug discovery because of the improving power or speed of the computer that led to advanced QM algorithm progress as well as a new application to address the shortcoming [70]. The popular method of fragment molecular orbital (FMO) offers a wide range of solutions where there are combined accuracy, speed, and the ability to characterize important interaction such as strength in kcal/mol as well as hydrophobic, electrostatic, and so on. In summary, FMO analyzed the length such as polarization, desolation, and interaction with the illustrated for a water dimer and protein-ligand complex [71].

3.2.4 Pharmacokinetic properties

Pharmacokinetics is the unique part of the drug design where the time course study is done through the mathematical characterization for absorption of drug, distribution, metabolism as well as excretion (ADME) [72]. Therefore, before the clinical trial, it is the advanced procedure to select a drug for the development and decision-maker by AMDE test [73]. As a result, it is safe and effective for a specific patient by decreasing toxicity and increasing efficacy in drug therapy. However, the central compartment of the human body was interconnected by a series of compartments reversibly on the base of pharmacokinetic [74]. Therefore, drugs enter each compartment and are distributed homogenously to display consistent kinetics. Hence, it is separated by a mathematical model where AMDE can differ in each compartment and help to predict drug metabolisms or actions [75]. Moreover, the central compartment received drug and entry on the body called absorption. The drug is distributed to the peripheral compartment after absorbing into the body and beginning the metabolic processes. Finally, the excretion of the drug from the body is in three ways such as hydrophilic molecules by the renal system, hydrophobic molecules by the biliary system, and volatile substances by the pulmonary system [76].

4. Immunoinformatic

4.1 Peptide design

In the drug discovery, peptides are not new, but it makes a choice drug candidate in the challenging situation with the collaboration of immunoinformatics. Immunoinformatics can be developed as natural endogenous scaffolds with familiar biological activities for solving challenging medical problems by it distinguishing characteristics such as the ability to act firstly, more specific, the minimum range of toxicity, and so on [77]. Approximately 55 therapeutic peptides have been approved for clinical trial through the regulatory agency [78]. Currently, many researchers have been working to solve various diseases through antimicrobial peptide design. The target of antimicrobial peptides has accelerated through the deep generative models and molecular dynamics. By utilizing the immunoinformatic approach, the researcher has developed 20 novel peptides that were validated through deep learning and high-throughput molecular simulation [79]. The peptides are not only used in broad-spectrum potency but also lead to multi-drug resistant strain and low toxicity. Immunoinformatic approaches help to observe peptide activity, selectivity, toxicity, ease of synthesis stability, etc. During the present situation of COVID-19, immunoinformatics help to identify peptide candidates from diverse viral sequences as shown in **Figure 4**, which can be utilized for vaccine design [80]. It is identified and designed from the motifs and subsequently a peptide library. As a result, strong binding affinities of peptides had happened with the main protease of SARS-CoC-2 as well as maintained stability and physiological condition observed by molecular dynamic simulation [81].

4.2 Vaccine design

Vaccine design is a very powerful tool for saving human life in the world broadly. The advancement of technology has been trigger to develop new strategies by the target and the structures of antibodies, hitting conserved epitopes and controlling the usage of antigenic variation [82]. It designed immunogens for provoking foreign responses because of no single or best solution of immune drugs design till now [83]. However, artificial intelligence and system biology together make an opportunity for avoiding inefficiencies and failures that help to classical vaccine development pipeline [84]. *In silico* vaccine design process has been selecting well fragment of virus protein [85], thereby finally leading to a final vaccine as shown in **Figure 4** [86].

However, in the vaccine design process, DeepVacPerd is an efficient tool that predicts the best vaccine subunit candidates with 30 subunit candidates from the various protein sequences within a second by replacing the predicted and selected with deep neural network architecture [87]. Therefore, it has become a promising of higher efficiencies for the vaccine design and test process. Furthermore, systems biology developed various tools by analyzing large data set through the complex modeling interaction between the individual interaction [88]. The omics disciplines such as genomics, proteomics, metabolisms, and so on produced a simulation of the immune response, identified response-specific signature, and assessed their predictive value through the basilar idea with the integration of high-throughput data [89]. Therefore, several programs and consortiums have performed by developing novel analytic tools that may integrate the information from omics.

4.3 Future perspective of vaccine

Personalized vaccine candidates are developed against a specific "targeted" to maintain an optimized outcome. Failure of the vaccine candidates can increase

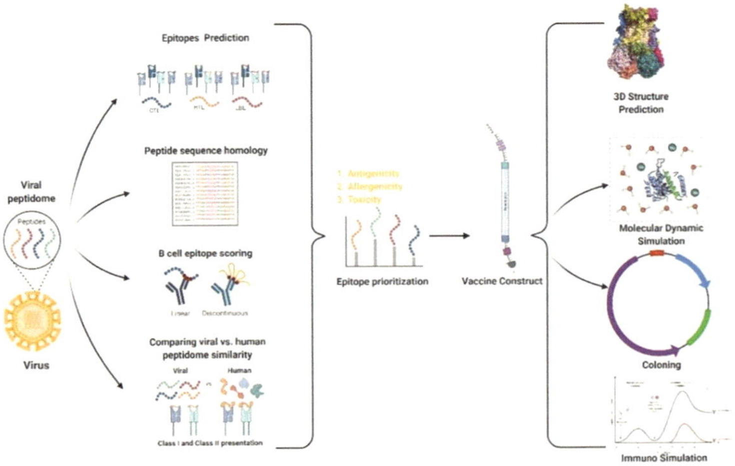

Figure 4.
Immunoinformatics aided identification of peptide candidates and procedure for designing multi-epitope vaccine by utilizing the peptide.

immunogenicity subsequently reactogenicity and adverse effects [90]. Therefore, the individual level, the gender level, the racial/ethnic level, and the subpopulation level should be considered during the personalized vaccine development process. Haplotype and polymorphism are mainly focused on the individual level selection as they can retard the formation of a protective immune response, where the gender level can determine the antibody tiger against a particular vaccine to males and females [91]. On the other hand, different human races or ethnic groups can show higher or lower immune responses to a specific vaccine candidate. Additionally, different interactions between host environmental, genetic, and some other factors may be influencing the vaccine immune responses; therefore, the subpopulation level should be also considered during vaccine design that can trigger an optimum immune response against a specific disease [92].

5. Conclusion

The study describes numerous computational tools that are widely used for drug and vaccine design against infectious viral diseases. However, improving ideas and methodologies can solve problems and provide system-level interconnected data. A promising idea accelerates the rational design of drug candidates that are used in the specific subfield. Here, we focused on computational methods that will help and provide a clear idea of modern drug and vaccine design approaches adequately.

Acknowledgements

The authors are in debt to King Abdulaziz University for their encouragements and unlimited support.

Conflict of interest

The authors declare no conflict of interest.

Author details

Mohammed Othman Aljahdali*, Mohammad Habibur Rahman Molla
and Foysal Ahammad
Faculty of Science, Department of Biological Sciences, King Abdulaziz University,
Jeddah, Saudi Arabia

*Address all correspondence to: moaljahdali@kau.edu.sa

References

[1] Shaw WR, Catteruccia F. Vector biology meets disease control: Using basic research to fight vector-borne diseases. Nature Microbiology. 2019;**4**(1):20-34. DOI: 10.1038/s41564-018-0214-7

[2] Rogers DJ, Packer MJ. Vector-borne diseases, models, and global change. Lancet. 1993;**342**(8882):1282-1284. DOI: 10.1016/0140-6736(93)92367-3

[3] Sainz Á, Roura X, Estrada-Peña A, Kohn B, Harrus S, Solano-Gallego L. Guideline for veterinary practitioners on canine ehrlichiosis and anaplasmosis in Europe. Parasites Vectors. 2015;**8**(1):1-20. DOI: 10.1186/S13071-015-0649-0

[4] Mourya DT, Yadav PD, Ullas PT, Bhardwaj SD, Sahay RR, Chadha MS, et al. Emerging/re-emerging viral diseases & new viruses on the Indian horizon. Indian Journal of Medical Research. 2019;**149**(4):447. DOI: 10.4103/IJMR.IJMR_1239_18

[5] Kruse H, Kirkemo A-M, Handeland K. Wildlife as source of zoonotic infections. Emerging Infectious Diseases. 2004; **10**(12):2067-2072. DOI: 10.3201/EID1012.040707

[6] Pulendran B, Arunachalam PS, O'Hagan DT. Emerging concepts in the science of vaccine adjuvants. Nature Reviews Drug Discovery. 2021;**20**(6):1. DOI: 10.1038/S41573-021-00163-Y

[7] Terry FE, Moise L, Martin RF, Torres M, Pilotte N, Williams SA, et al. Time for T? Immunoinformatics addresses vaccine design for neglected tropical and emerging infectious diseases. Expert Review of Vaccines. 2015;**14**(1):21-35. DOI: 10.1586/14760584.2015.955478

[8] V'kovski P, Kratzel A, Steiner S, Stalder H, Thiel V. Coronavirus biology and replication: Implications for SARS-CoV-2. Nature Reviews Microbiology. 2020;**19**(3):155-170. DOI: 10.1038/s41579-020-00468-6

[9] Modrow S, Falke D, Truyen U, Schätzl H. Viruses with single-stranded, positive-sense RNA genomes. Molecular Virology. 2013:185-349. DOI: 10.1007/978-3-642-20718-1_14

[10] Khan T, Lawerence AJ, Azad I, Raza S, Joshi S, Khan AR. Computational drug designing and prediction of important parameters using *in silico* methods- A review. Current Computer-Aided Drug Design. 2019;**15**(5):384-397. DOI: 10.2174/1573399815666190326120006

[11] Sweiti H, Wiegand F, Bug C, Vogel M, Lavie F, Winiger-Candolfi I, et al. Physicians in the pharmaceutical industry: Their roles, motivations, and perspectives. Drug Discovery Today. 2019;**24**(9):1865-1870. DOI: 10.1016/J.DRUDIS.2019.05.021

[12] Rifaioglu AS, Atas H, Martin MJ, Cetin-Atalay R, Atalay V, Doğan T. Recent applications of deep learning and machine intelligence on *in silico* drug discovery: Methods, tools and databases. Briefings in Bioinformatics. 2019;**20**(5):1878-1912. DOI: 10.1093/BIB/BBY061

[13] Furuse Y. Analysis of research intensity on infectious disease by disease burden reveals which infectious diseases are neglected by researchers. Proceedings of the National Academy of Science of the United States of America. 2019;**116**(2):478-483. DOI: 10.1073/PNAS.1814484116

[14] Dasaraju PV, Liu C. Infections of the Respiratory System. In: Baron S, editor.

Medical Microbiology. 4th ed. Galveston (TX): University of Texas Medical Branch at Galveston; 1996

[15] Relman DA, Lipsitch M. Microbiome as a tool and a target in the effort to address antimicrobial resistance. Proceedings of the National Academy of Sciences of the United States of America. 2018;**115**(51):12902-12910. DOI: 10.1073/PNAS.1717163115

[16] Janeway CA Jr, Travers P, Walport M, Shlomchik MJ. Infectious Agents and How They cause Disease. 5th ed. New York: Garland Science; 2001. Available from: https://www.ncbi.nlm.nih.gov/books/NBK27114/ [Accessed: October 07, 2021]

[17] Edemekong PF, Huang B. Epidemiology of prevention of communicable diseases. In: StatPearls [Internet]. Treasure Island (FL): StatPearls Publishing; Jan 2021

[18] Funk S, Gilad E, Watkins C, Jansen VA. The spread of awareness and its impact on epidemic outbreaks. Proceedings of the National Academy of Sciences of the United States of America. 2009;**106**(16):6872-6877. DOI: 10.1073/pnas.0810762106

[19] Rohr JR, Barrett CB, Civitello DJ, Craft ME, Delius B, GA DL, et al. Emerging human infectious diseases and the links to global food production. Nature Sustainability. 2019;**2**(6):445-456. DOI: 10.1038/s41893-019-0293-3

[20] Greger M. The human/animal interface: Emergence and resurgence of zoonotic infectious diseases. Critical Reviews in Microbiology. 2007;**33**(4):243-299. DOI: 10.1080/10408410701647594

[21] Smith KF, Goldberg M, Rosenthal S, Carlson L, Chen J, Chen C, et al. Global rise in human infectious disease outbreaks. Journal of the Royal Society Interface. 2014;**11**(101):20140950. DOI: 10.1098/RSIF.2014.0950

[22] Bhutta ZA, Sommerfeld J, Lassi ZS, Salam RA, Das JK. Global burden, distribution, and interventions for infectious diseases of poverty. Infectious Diseases of Poverty. 2014;**3**(1):1-7. DOI: 10.1186/2049-9957-3-21

[23] Alghamdi AA. Impact of the COVID-19 pandemic on the social and educational aspects of Saudi university students' lives. PLoS One. 2021;**16**(4):e0250026. DOI: 10.1371/JOURNAL.PONE.0250026

[24] Mathers CD, Bernard C, Iburg KM, Inoue M, Ma Fat D, Shibuya K, et al. Global Burden of Disease in 2002: Data sources, methods and results [Internet]. 2003. Available from: www.who.int/evidence/bod [Accessed: October 07, 2021]

[25] Ung L, Chodosh J. Foundational concepts in the biology of bacterial keratitis. Experimental Eye Research. 2021;**209**:108647. DOI: 10.1016/J.EXER.2021.108647

[26] Mourya DT, Yadav PD, Ullas PT, Bhardwaj SD, Sahay RR, Chadha MS, et al. Emerging/re-emerging viral diseases & new viruses on the Indian horizon. Indian Journal of Medical Research. 2019;**149**(4):447-467. DOI: 10.4103/IJMR.IJMR_1239_18

[27] Jones KE, Patel NG, Levy MA, Storeygard A, Balk D, Gittleman JL, et al. Global trends in emerging infectious diseases. Nature. 2008;**451**(7181):990. DOI: 10.1038/NATURE06536

[28] Li H, Yang Y, Hong W, Huang M, Wu M, Zhao X. Applications of genome editing technology in the targeted therapy of human diseases: Mechanisms, advances and prospects. Signal Transduction and

Targeted Therapy. 2020;**5**(1):1-23. DOI: 10.1038/s41392-019-0089-y

[29] Pinter-Wollman N, Jelić A, Wells NM. The impact of the built environment on health behaviours and disease transmission in social systems. Philosophical Transactions of the Royal Society B Biological Sciences. 2018;**373**(1753). DOI: 10.1098/RSTB.2017.0245

[30] Gomez-Lus R, Clavel A, Castillo J, Seral C, Rubio C. Emerging and reemerging pathogens. International Journal of Antimicrobial Agents. 2000; **16**(3):335-339. DOI: 10.1016/S0924-8579(00)00261-2

[31] Weaver SC, Costa F, Garcia-Blanco MA, Ko AI, Ribeiro GS, Saade G, et al. Zika virus: History, emergence, biology, and prospects for control. Antiviral Research. 2016;**130**:69. DOI: 10.1016/J. ANTIVIRAL.2016.03.010

[32] Meyding-Lamadé U, Craemer E, Schnitzler P. Emerging and re-emerging viruses affecting the nervous system. Neurological Research and Practice. 2019;**1**(1):1-9. DOI: 10.1186/S42466-019-0020-6

[33] Dabbu Kumar J, Jian L, Rong H, Hua Z. Emerging and reemerging human viral diseases. Annals of Microbiology and Research. 2018;**2**(1):31-44. DOI: 10.36959/958/567

[34] Bloom DE, Cadarette D. Infectious disease threats in the twenty-first century: Strengthening the global response. Frontiers in Immunology. 2019;**10**:549. DOI: 10.3389/FIMMU.2019.00549

[35] Feldman C, Shaddock E. Epidemiology of lower respiratory tract infections in adults. Expert Review of Respiratory Medicine. 2019;**13**(1):63-77. DOI: 10.1080/17476348.2019.1555040

[36] Morse SS. Factors in the emergence of infectious diseases. Emerging Infectious Diseases. 1995;**1**(1):7-15. DOI: 10.3201/EID0101.950102

[37] Schneider UA, Havlik P, Schmid E, Valin H, Mosnier A, Obersteiner M, et al. Impacts of population growth, economic development, and technical change on global food production and consumption. Agricultural Systems. 2011;**104**(2):204-215. DOI: 10.1016/J. AGSY.2010.11.003

[38] Reed KD. Respiratory tract infections: A clinical approach. Molecular Medical Microbiology. 2015;**3**:1499-1506. DOI: 10.1016/B978-0-12-397169-2.00084-6

[39] Ogilvie M. Molecular techniques should not now replace cell culture in diagnostic virology laboratories. Reviews in Medical Virology. 2001;**11**(6):351-354. DOI: 10.1002/RMV.335

[40] Zampieri F. The impact of modern medicine on human evolution. In: Tibayrene M, Ayala FJ, editors. On Human Nature Biology, Psychology, Ethics, Politics, and Religion. Academic Press; 2017. pp. 707-727. DOI: 10.1016/B978-0-12-420190-3.00043-0. Available from: https://www.semanticscholar.org/paper/The-Impact-of-Modern-Medicine-on-Human-Evolution-Zampieri/af39aabd82bbeace3588e98cfb23538e77946e66

[41] Morens DM, Folkers GK, Fauci AS. The challenge of emerging and re-emerging infectious diseases. Nature. 2004;**430**(6996):242-249. DOI: 10.1038/nature02759

[42] Plotkin BJ, Kimball AM. Designing an international policy and legal framework for the control of emerging infectious diseases: First steps. Emerging Infectious Diseases. 1997;3(1):1-9. DOI: 10.3201/EID0301.970101

[43] Blastland M, Freeman ALJ, van der Linden S, Marteau TM, Spiegelhalter D. Five rules for evidence communication. Nature. 2020;**587**(7834):362-364. DOI: 10.1038/D41586-020-03189-1

[44] Araj R, Alqasrawi S, Samy S, Alwahdanee G, Waldi J, Mofleh J, et al. Preventing emerging and re-emerging infections in the eastern mediterranean region: Gaps, challenges, and priorities. JMIR Public Health and Surveillance. 2019;**5**(4):e14348. DOI: 10.2196/14348

[45] Hughes JM, Wilson ME, Pike BL, Saylors KE, Fair JN, LeBreton M, et al. The origin and prevention of pandemics. Clinical Infectious Diseases. 2010;50(12):1636-1640. DOI: 10.1086/652860

[46] Mahady GB. Medicinal plants for the prevention and treatment of bacterial infections. Current Pharmaceutical Design. 2005;**11**(19):2405-2427. DOI: 10.2174/1381612054367481

[47] Aljahdali MO, Molla MHR, Ahammad F. Compounds identified from marine mangrove plant (*Avicennia alba*) as potential antiviral drug candidates against WDSV, an in-silico approach. Marine Drugs. 2021;**19**(5):253. DOI: 10.3390/MD19050253

[48] Wang L, Wang Y, Jin S, Wu Z, Chin DP, Koplan JP, et al. Emergence and control of infectious diseases in China. The Lancet. 2008;**372**(9649):1598-1605. DOI: 10.1016/S0140-6736(08)61365-3

[49] Mukherjee S. Emerging infectious diseases: Epidemiological perspective. Indian Journal of Dermatology. Sep. 2017;**62**(5):459-467. DOI: 10.4103/IJD.IJD_379_17

[50] Achan J, Talisuna AO, Erhart A, Yeka A, Tibenderana JK, Baliraine FN, et al. Quinine, an old anti-malarial drug in a modern world: Role in the treatment of malaria. Malaria Journal. 2011;**10**:144. DOI: 10.1186/1475-2875-10-144

[51] Kutlushina A, Khakimova A, Madzhidov T, Polishchuk P. Ligand-based pharmacophore modeling using novel 3D pharmacophore signatures. Molecules. 2018;**23**(12):3094. DOI: 10.3390/MOLECULES23123094

[52] Duerr TJ, Comellas E, Jeon EK, Farkas JE, Joetzjer M, Garnier J, et al. 3D visualization of macromolecule synthesis. Elife. 2020;**9**:e60354. DOI: 10.1101/2020.06.24.169300

[53] Yang SY. Pharmacophore modeling and applications in drug discovery: Challenges and recent advances. Drug Discovery Today. 2010;**15**(11-12):444-450. DOI: 10.1016/J.DRUDIS.2010.03.013

[54] Ferreira LG, Dos Santos RN, Oliva G, Andricopulo AD. Molecular docking and structure-based drug design strategies. Molecules. 2015;**20**(7):13384-13421. DOI: 10.3390/MOLECULES200713384

[55] Wang W, Ye Z, Gao H, Ouyang D. Computational pharmaceutics - A new paradigm of drug delivery. Journal of Controlled Release. 2021;**338**:119-136. DOI: 10.1016/J.JCONREL.2021.08.030

[56] Sousa SF, Fernandes PA, Ramos MJ. Protein-ligand docking: Current status and future challenges. Proteins. 2006;**65**(1):15-26. DOI: 10.1002/PROT.21082

[57] Khanam H, Ali A, Asif M, Shamsuzzaman. Neurodegenerative diseases linked to misfolded proteins and their therapeutic approaches: A review. European Journal of Medicinal Chemistry. 2016;**124**:1121-1141. DOI: 10.1016/J.EJMECH.2016.08.006

[58] Sliwoski G, Kothiwale S, Meiler J, Lowe EW Jr. Computational methods

in drug discovery. Pharmacological Reviews. 2014;**66**(1):334. DOI: 10.1124/PR.112.007336

[59] Atanasov AG, Waltenberger B, Pferschy-Wenzig E-M, Linder T, Wawrosch C, Uhrin P, et al. Discovery and resupply of pharmacologically active plant-derived natural products: A review. Biotechnology Advances. 2015;**33**(8):1582-1614. DOI: 10.1016/j.biotechadv.2015.08.001

[60] Mori T, Miyashita N, Im W, Feig M, Sugita Y. Molecular dynamics simulations of biological membranes and membrane proteins using enhanced conformational sampling algorithms. Biochimica et Biophysica Acta (BBA) - Biomembranes. 2016;**1858**(7):1635-1651. DOI: 10.1016/J.BBAMEM.2015.12.032

[61] Pritchett DB, Seeburg PH. The role of molecular biology in drug discovery and design. In: Harris TJR, editor. Protein Production by Biotechnology. Boston: Springer; 1990. pp. 181-190. DOI: 10.1007/978-1-4613-1565-0_14

[62] Swegat W, Schlitter J, Krüger P, Wollmer A. MD simulation of protein-ligand interaction: Formation and dissociation of an insulin-phenol complex. Biophysical Journal. 2003;**84**(3):1493-1506. DOI: 10.1016/S0006-3495(03)74962-5

[63] Lee S, Bhattacharya S, Tate CG, Grisshammer R, Vaidehi N. Structural dynamics and thermostabilization of neurotensin receptor 1. The Journal of Physical Chemistry B. 2015;**119**(15):4917-4928. DOI: 10.1021/JP510735F

[64] González MA. Force fields and molecular dynamics simulations. Collection SFN. 2011;**12**:169-200. DOI: 10.1051/sfn/201112009

[65] Lesiuk M. Implementation of the coupled-cluster method with single, double, and triple excitations using tensor decompositions. Journal of Chemical Theory and Computation. 2019;**16**(1):453-467. DOI: 10.1021/ACS.JCTC.9B00985

[66] Arodola OA, Soliman ME. Quantum mechanics implementation in drug-design workflows: Does it really help? Drug Design, Development and Therapy. 2017;**11**:2551-2564. DOI: 10.2147/DDDT.S126344

[67] Taylor D. The pharmaceutical industry and the future of drug development. Issues in Environmental Science and Technology. 2015;**2016**(41):1-33. DOI: 10.1039/9781782622345-00001

[68] Lonsdale R, Fort RM, Rydberg P, Harvey JN, Mulholland AJ. Quantum mechanics/molecular mechanics modeling of drug metabolism: Mexiletine N-hydroxylation by cytochrome P450 1A2. Chemical Research in Toxicology. 2016;**29**(6):963-971. DOI: 10.1021/ACS.CHEMRESTOX.5B00514

[69] Kalaszi A, Imre G, Jakli I, Farkas O. Identification of the bioactive conformation for mucin epitope peptides. Journal of Molecular Structure: THEOCHEM. 2007;**823**(1-3):16-27. DOI: 10.1016/J.THEOCHEM.2007.08.016

[70] Salo-Ahen OMH, Alanko I, Bhadane R, Bonvin AMJJ, Honorato RV, Hossain S, et al. Molecular dynamics simulations in drug discovery and pharmaceutical development. Process. 2021;**9**(1):71. DOI: 10.3390/PR9010071

[71] Fedorov DG, Nagata T, Kitaura K. Exploring chemistry with the fragment molecular orbital method. Physical Chemistry Chemical Physics. 2012;**14**(21):7562-7577. DOI: 10.1039/C2CP23784A

[72] Wu F, Zhou Y, Li L, Shen X, Chen G, Wang X, et al. Computational

approaches in preclinical studies on drug discovery and development. Frontiers in Chemistry. 2020;**8**:726. DOI: 10.3389/fchem.2020.00726

[73] Sutton RT, Pincock D, Baumgart DC, Sadowski DC, Fedorak RN, Kroeker KI. An overview of clinical decision support systems: Benefits, risks, and strategies for success. npj Digital Medicine. 2020;**3**(1):1-10. DOI: 10.1038/s41746-020-0221-y

[74] Kok-Yong S, Lawrence L. Drug Distribution and Drug Elimination. Basic Pharmacokinetic Concepts and Some Clinical Applications. London: IntechOpen; 2015. DOI: 10.5772/59929

[75] Vendel E, Rottschäfer V, de Lange ECM. The need for mathematical modelling of spatial drug distribution within the brain. Fluids and Barriers of the CNS. 2019;**16**(1):1-33. DOI: 10.1186/S12987-019-0133-X

[76] Prabu SL, Suriyaprakash TNK, Ruckmani K, Thirumurugan R. Biopharmaceutics and Pharmacokinetics. Basic Pharmacokinetic Concepts and Some Clinical Applications. IntechOpen; 2015. DOI: 10.5772/61160. Available from: https://www.intechopen.com/chapters/48805

[77] Henninot A, Collins JC, Nuss JM. The current state of peptide drug discovery: Back to the future? Journal of Medicinal Chemistry. 2017;**61**(4):1382-1414. DOI: 10.1021/ACS.JMEDCHEM.7B00318

[78] Lau JL, Dunn MK. Therapeutic peptides: Historical perspectives, current development trends, and future directions. Bioorganic & Medicinal Chemistry. 2018;**26**(10):2700-2707. DOI: 10.1016/J.BMC.2017.06.052

[79] Zharkova MS, Orlov DS, Golubeva OY, Chakchir OB, Eliseev IE, Grinchuk TM, et al. Application of antimicrobial peptides of the innate immune system in combination with conventional antibiotics—A novel way to combat antibiotic resistance? Frontiers in Cellular and Infection Microbiology. 2019;**9**:128. DOI: 10.3389/FCIMB.2019.00128

[80] Debnath S, Barnaby DP, Coppa K, Makhnevich A, Kim EJ, Chatterjee S, et al. Machine learning to assist clinical decision-making during the COVID-19 pandemic. Bioelectronic Medicine. 2020;**6**(1):1-8. DOI: 10.1186/S42234-020-00050-8

[81] Eichmann M, de Ru A, van Veelen PA, Peakman M, Kronenberg-Versteeg D. Identification and characterisation of peptide binding motifs of six autoimmune disease-associated human leukocyte antigen-class I molecules including HLA-B*39:06. Tissue Antigens. 2014;**84**(4):378-388. DOI: 10.1111/TAN.12413

[82] Curtiss R. Expert review of vaccines vaccine design: Innovative approaches and novel strategies. Expert Review Vaccines. 2011;**10**(10):1385-1387. DOI: 10.1586/erv.11.114

[83] De Groot AS, Moise L, Terry F, Guiterrez AH, Hindocha P, Richard G, et al. Better epitope discovery, precision immune engineering, and accelerated vaccine design using immunoinformatics tools. Frontiers in Immunology. 2020;**11**: 442. DOI: 10.3389/FIMMU.2020.00442

[84] Urrutia-Baca VH, Gomez-Flores R, De La Garza-Ramos MA, Tamez-Guerra P, Lucio-Sauceda DG, Rodríguez-padilla MC. Immunoinformatics approach to design a novel epitope-based oral vaccine against *Helicobacter pylori*. Journal of Computational Biology. 2019;**26**(10):1177-1190. DOI: 10.1089/CMB.2019.0062

[85] Ali SA, Almofti YA, Khoubieb KA. Immunoinformatics approach for

multiepitopes vaccine prediction against glycoprotein B of avian infectious laryngotracheitis virus. Advances in Bioinformatics. 2019;**2019**:1270485. DOI: 10.1155/2019/1270485

[86] Russo G, Reche P, Pennisi M, Pappalardo F. The combination of artificial intelligence and systems biology for intelligent vaccine design. Expert Opinion on Drug Discovery. 2020;**15**:11, 1267-1281. DOI: 10.1080/17460441.2020.1791076

[87] Arora P, Kumar H, Panigrahi BK. Prediction and analysis of COVID-19 positive cases using deep learning models: A descriptive case study of India. Chaos, Solitons & Fractals. 2020;**139**:110017. DOI: 10.1016/J.CHAOS.2020.110017

[88] Nazem-Bokaee H, Hom EFY, Warden AC, Mathews S, Gueidan C. Towards a systems biology approach to understanding the lichen symbiosis: Opportunities and challenges of implementing network modelling. Frontiers in Microbiology. 2021;**12**:1028. DOI: 10.3389/FMICB.2021.667864

[89] Jerez CA. The use of genomics, proteomics and other OMICS technologies for the global understanding of biomining microorganisms. Hydrometallurgy. 2008;**94**(1-4):162-169. DOI: 10.1016/J.HYDROMET.2008.05.032

[90] Oli AN, Obialor WO, Ifeanyichukwu MO, Odimegwu DC, Okoyeh JN, Emechebe GO, et al. Immunoinformatics and vaccine development: An overview. Immunotargets and Therapy. 2020;**9**:13-30. DOI: 10.2147/ITT.S241064

[91] Filatov DA, Charlesworth D. DNA polymorphism, haplotype structure and balancing selection in the Leavenworthia PgiC locus. Genetics. 1999;**153**(3):1423-1434

[92] Huang T, Shu Y, Cai Y-D. Genetic differences among ethnic groups. BMC Genomics. 2015;**16**(1):1-10. DOI: 10.1186/S12864-015-2328-0

Chapter 5

Reprofiling of Octogenarian Antiviral Agent: A New Avenue Venture to Discover Viral Infection

Nikhat Farhana, Mohammed Gulzar Ahmed, Mohammed Asif Iqbal, Nishmitha Gretta D'Souza, Sudhina Makuttan, Natasha Naval Aggarwal and Abdul Rahamanulla

Abstract

Identification of a new drug molecule to a new target, specifically viral, bacterial, and fungal infection, is the prime focus of time immortal. The tridiagonal practice of drug discovery for emerging viral infection turned out to be a new venture to combat the morbidly and mortality of recent pandemics due to viral, bacterial, fungal, infection and infestation, the emerging number of viral infections day by day, the targeted therapy with the gap in assessment lead to reprofiling or repositioning available FDA-approved formulation give promising drug candidate for various infection specifically the current scenario of antiviral drug-reprofiling through drug designing approach, the emergence of resistance to existing antiviral drugs and re-emerging viral infections are the greatest challenges in antiviral drug discovery. The reprofiling approach is a worthy strategy to get the potent antiviral in brief span of time to overcome the challenges in antiviral therapy. The present chapter will be another representing the most promising results of reprofiling (Repositioning or repurposing) approach in the treatment of various infectious diseases.

Keywords: antiviral, drug-resistance, re-emerging, viral infection, fungal infection, bacterial infection

1. Introduction

Drug Repurposing, repositioning and reprofiling is trending initiative adopted by the researcher to identify the new target with existing drug molecule, the chemotherapeutic intervention of antiviral drugs discovery, frequently unsynchronized with development and licensing of the new drug, diseased caused by the virous is not an exceptional way of treating with antiviral agents. COVID-19 was turnout to be the major pandemic of the 21st century which is highly contagious, with more the 200 million cases and 4.5 million deaths worldwide to date, this pandemic created wreaked havoc in society with immense human suffering. In a race against time to stop the spread of the disease. Contemporaneous endeavor scientific research community put forth several active molecules which inhibit the SARS-CoV-2 infection within period. Based on the background of literature report viral entry and replication within the host of the cell involves multiple molecular factors associated with the host and virous both, among this important one is a Main protease (M^{pro}), which is also referred to as 3C-like protease (3C-L^{pro}). M^{pro} cleavage of the viral polyprotein PP1ab at 11 discrete sites (polyproteins encoded with Leu-Gly-fl-Ser/Gly/Ala as motif cleavage). After cleavage it released non-structural protein from replicase complex, which is essential for viral replication, the proteolytic cleavage inhibition can prevent SARS-CoV-2 replication inside the host cell, hence in antiviral drug discovery, the M^{pro} is a prime target against SARS-CoV-2. Beginning of the first case of COVID-19, intensive literature reviled that M^{pro} is prime suspect targeted with several drug candidates which include both ab initio designed as well as repositioning of drugs. Notable recent discovery reports on repositioning approach with electrophilic and noncovalent fragment screening against M^{pro} in combination with Mass spectrometry and X-ray crystallography found to be an excellent technique to figure out the active site as well as dimerization interface, several potent small-molecule inhibitors of SARS-CoV-2 M^{pro} were predicted in a recent year since the beginning of this pandemic outbreak with all-inclusive nature of work vindicated by the discovery of both mentioned above in the paragraph.

However, to be noted here, 12 antiviral drugs were approved by FDA in the USA till date, among these 8 are used to treat hepatitis C virus (HCV)-related pathologies and 2 are in the combination of anti-human immunodeficiency virus (HIV) agents. WHO

S.NO	PRECEDENCE	PITFALLS
1	Low cost and less time-consuming (essential for the development of drugs to treat neglected diseases)	Target identification can be circuitous, and identified drugs may show poly-pharmacology
2	Possibility to skip preclinical trials (no animal studies) and to directly enter phase 2 clinical trials	Due to the high doses employed ill the screenings, toxic drugs can be initially misidentified as active
3	Potential for combination strategies with the possibility to delay or reduce resistance associated with monotherapy	Effective concentrations are often higher than the plasma levels achievable in humans
4	Often analogy (together with pharmacological information) are already available for testing	Medicinal chemistry to design more potent analogy is not applicable without losing repurposing potential
5	Academic/small laboratories can be determinant in the drug-discovery process	Identified drugs are often under intellectual property and/or programs that make them unavailable or unattractive for other pharmaceutical companies that could take over the further development and costs of clinical trials
6	Formulations and manufacturing chains are already established for the large-scale production (launching costs are avoided)	

Table 1.
Precedence and pitfalls of a drug repurposing approach for antiviral drug discovery.

S.No	Library (Vendor)	Description
1	SCREEN-WELL FDA-Approved drugs Library (Enzo Life Sciences)	774 approved drugs
2	Library Of Pharmacologically Active Compounds (LOPAC, Sigma-Aldrich)	1280 bioactive compounds including FDA-approved drugs
3	Bioactive Compound Library (Selleck Chemicals)	>2000 bioactive compounds including FDA-approved drugs
4	Prestwick Library	1280 bioactive compounds including FDA-approved drugs and candidate drugs
5	Spectrum Collection (Micro-source)	2320–2560 bioactive compounds including FDA-approved drugs
6	UCSF Small Molecule Discovery Centre Library	2177 bioactive compounds including FDA-approved drugs
7	National Institute of Health (NIH) Clinical Collection Library and Chemical Genomics Centre (NCCGC)	>7600 bioactive compounds including FDA-approved drugs and candidate drugs

Table 2.
Small-molecule libraries used in antiviral drug repurposing.

dealing with the re-emerging viruses responsible for pandemic potential and alarming outbreak in recent years, which was still lacking specific treatment, such as Zika virus (ZIKV), Ebola Virus (EBOV), Middle East respiratory syndrome coronavirus (MERS-CoV), COVID-19, delta virus and nowadays the popular one OMICRON. The recent advancement in controlling this viral pathogen, drug discovery in the drug repurposing approach emerged as giving the old drug to new symptoms which unlock the unidentified molecular pathway with the target of intervention. Basically, this strategy was adopted to combat viral infectious disease, by integrating with combination with computational methods (in silico screening, mining of database with transcriptomic profile, etc. (**Tables 1** and **2**), and collective screening of small bioactive molecules.

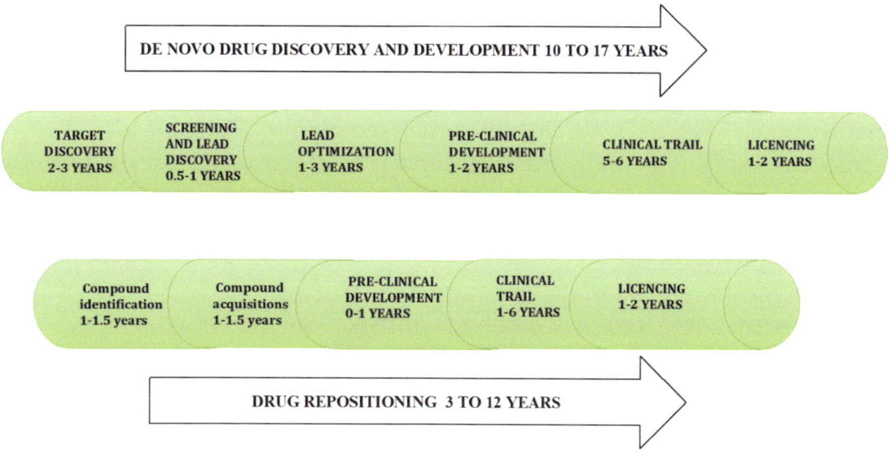

Figure 1.
DD and DR pathway.

Unquestionably a new drug development, in order to search for the lead molecule or pathway with biological screening that could be recycled against the viral pathogen, will be a competitive economic advantage, on the level of fundamental needs, indeed repurposed drugs quickly enter the clinical trial especially in case of viral disease lacking specified treatment (**Figure 1**) [1].

DR represents the constant source, to update and upgrade, cognition, in viral biology with available antiviral molecules hidden potentiality, which comes out as a tool to unlock the molecular mechanisms of virous replication and pathogenesis. No doubt, DR explore unidentified cellular pathway, turning them into target for the unexplored therapeutic strategy to available molecules which were not even under clinical trial. This book chapter is a unique and only compact reference to the researcher who are involved in reprofiling existing drugs, with promising drugs, meaningful results, and conclusions on the repurposing of antiviral drugs discovery [2].

2. Identification of antiviral drug repurposing

The drug repurposing approach is the process of finding new indications for existing FDA-approved drugs, is promising alternative to accelerate the process of drug development for infectious diseases and many other disorders and diseases, DR can be pursued by three possible strategies which are as follows.

Pre-clinical studies: This study was conducted in-vitro or in-vivo animal models before proceeding towards the clinical studies in the patient, whether healthy or sick. This also includes in silico in-vitro such as receptor-binding sassy to identify drug ligands and studies using cell line or tissue excised from animal or human representative of the specific disease, to examine how biological milieus of varying complexity response to the drug. In-vivo is also conduct in animals to test the biological parameters by sacrificing an animal for histological behaviors in rats or mice, here the available preclinical model can be used for repurposing to generate a hypothesis, this study is a preliminary study which is the base for setting up the clinical studies.

Clinical studies: Ranging from single-arm open-label **trial** to randomized controlled trial (RCTs) provides information on drug tolerance and efficacy, the notable interplay between regulatory and government bodies and research conducting clinical trial, as such entity have role in regulating clinical trial.

Observational studies: This study provides evidence to the findings it relays on data that is existing or data collected quickly in a prospective manner using previously established data system and conducted rapidly. The main aim of observational study evidence generation concerned drugs which use off-label for COVID-19 for example retrospective observational studies during the pandemic in Italy hospital. The limitation of observational studies is often based on secondary data. Refer **Figure 2**.

- **Same target-new virus:** These kinds of antiviral agents are having target-specific cellular function/pathway found to possess activity against other viruses (relies on homology and common enzymatic features of viral replication process).

1. Example-RNA-polymerize inhibitors such Favipiravir and sofosuvir. (Approved drug to treat influenza and HCV infection) this shows repurposing potential against EBOV and ZIKA

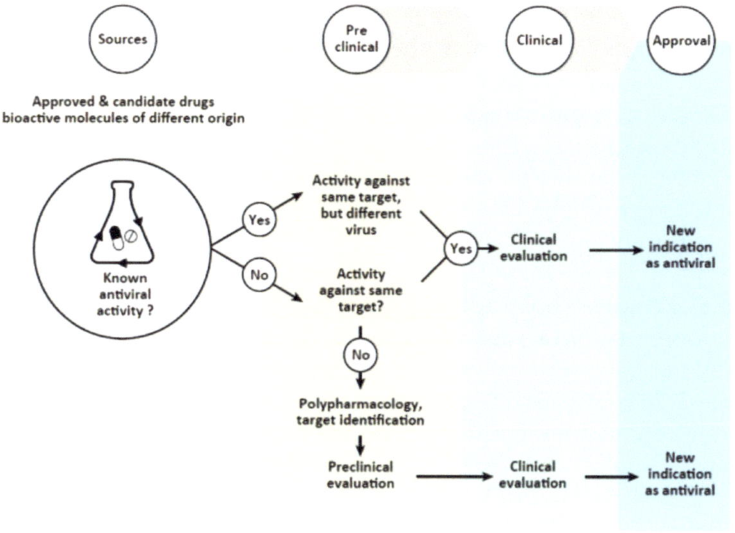

Figure 2.
FDA-approved formulation proceeds through 3- strategy steps, identified molecule-based target similarity hypothesis on viral pathway, absence of activity shows poly-pharmacology interference with different function (cellular or viral).

2. Example- Cellular endocytic pathway to enter the host cell (Chloroquine), interferes with the late-stage entry process of viruses (Filoviruses & coronaviruses)

- **Same target-new indication**: Pharmacological target essential in the pathogenesis of viral infection is modulated by approved drugs.

Example-1: Here approved drugs were exploited as an antiviral therapeutic agent (new indication).

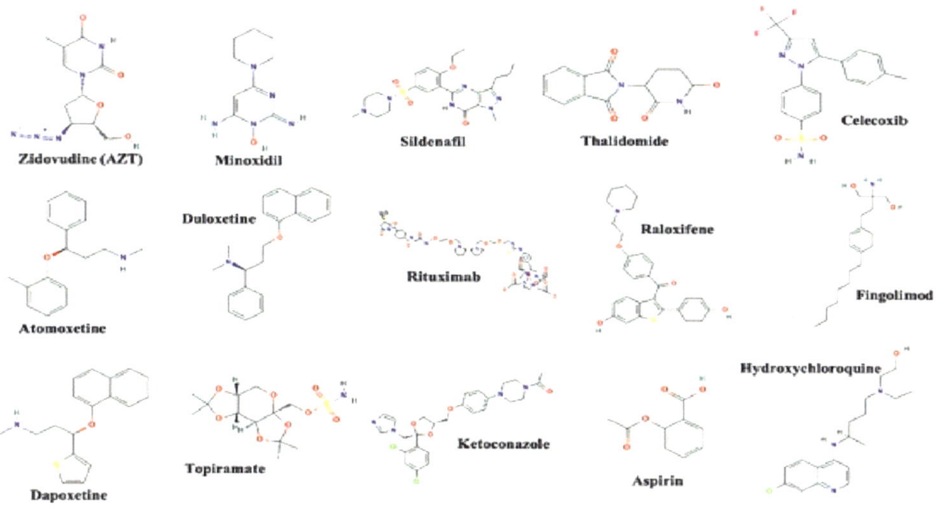

Figure 3.
FDA-approved multiply-acting drugs.

Example-2: Anticancer agents such as imatinib were found to be active against coronaviruses by inhibiting cellular Abelson (ABL) kinase

- **New target- new indication:** Here approved drugs were established with bioactivity in specific pathway/mechanism with new molecular target [Poly-Pharmacology (ability of approved drugs or pharmaceutical molecule to act on multiple targets might be toxicity or side effect) represent important opportunity to repurposing] molecule essential for virus replication.

Example-1: Antimicrobial agent which found to have targeted virus-infected cells as well as inhibition of viral replication (teicoplanin, ivermectin, itraconazole, and niazoxanide).

Example-2: Recently used SARS-CoV-2 and HIV drug to combat morbidity and mortality causes of viruses' outbreak examples of drugs are given (**Figure 3**).

Mentioned chemical structures are promising re-profiled candidates of FDA-approved drugs with its multiple actions, [3].

3. Repurposing in Zikv virus and other Flaviviruses infection

It was a mosquito-borne flavivirus, associated with several birth defects which are associated with infant neurological disorder (Gullain-Barre syndrome and other) and severe congenital defects in Newbern (microcephaly and ophthalmological alteration) such infection occurs during pregnancy. These viruses are capable of spreading both vertical (transplacental) and sexual, this infection is prime concerned for globule and public health, neither specific antiviral treatment nor a vaccine to counteract ZIKV diffusion is available to date. Henceforth FDA-approved drug repurposing camping started by WHO.

The library of 774 FDA-approved immunosuppressant drugs candidates were tested on HuH-7 hepatocytes cell-cultured strains isolated from ZIKV, among which 24 candidates showed potent anti-ZIKV activity which inhibits the ZIKV replication,

Drugs:

- Ivermectin, mycophenolic acid, daptomycin (Cross placenta barrier). FDA-approved Anthelmintics such as Niclosamide, Macrolide Azithromycin (Category B used during pregnancy).

- The structural based in silico screening followed by in-vitro and in-vivo leads to the identification of potent anti-ZIKV antibiotics such as Novobiocin, niclosamide, nanchangmycin, natural alkaloidal compound like hippeastrine hydrobromide (HH) and temoporfin which inhibits NS3/NS2B protease.

- Sofobuvrin Anti-HCV and anti-alzheimer's also reprofiled for Anti-ZIKV infection and to date, none of this are evaluated for the clinical trial [4].

3.1 Repurposing in Ebola virus infection

EBOV was discovered in the late 1970s but the outbreak was in 2014-2016 was an alarming period due to its size and spread, the cases were reported internationally in

S.NO	COMPOUND	STATUS/INDICATION	VIRUS	EXPERIMENTAL MODEL	TARGET
	FDA-Approved Synthetic drug candidates with repurposing potentials				
1.	Mycophenolic acid	Approved/immunomodulator	ZIKV	Infected cells in vitro	Undetermined
2.	Daptomycin	Approved/antibacterial	ZIKV	Infected cells in vitro	Undetermined
3.	Niclosamide	Approved/antiparasitic	ZIKV	Infected cells in vitro	ND and NS2B/NS3 protease
4.	Azithromycin	Approved/antibacterial	ZIKV	Infected cells in vitro	Undetermined
5.	Novobiocin	Approved/antibacterial	ZIKV	Infected cells in vitro mouse model	NS2B/NS3 protease
6.	Nanchangmycin	Investigational	ZIKV	Infected cells in vitro, mouse neuron–glia ex vivo cultures	Virus entry
7.	Hippeastrine hydrobromide	Investigational	ZIKV	Infected cells in vitro, organoids, mouse model	Undetermined
8.	Sofosbuvir	Approved/antiviral	ZIKV	Infected cells in vitro, mouse model	NS5 RNA polymerase
9.	Ribavirin	Approved/antiviral	ZIKV	Infected cells in vitro, mouse model	NS5 RNA polymerase
10.	Chloroquine	Approved/antimalarial	ZIKV, –	Infected cells in vitro, mouse model of vertical transmission	Undetermined
			MERS-CoV SARS- CoV	Infected cells in vitro	Undetermined
11.	Memantine	Approved/treatment of Alzheimer's disease	ZIKV	Primary neurons in vitro, mouse model	Undetermined
12.	Prochlorperazine	Approved/antiemetic	DENV	Infected cells in vitro, mouse model	Entry?
13.	Chlorcyclizine	Approved/antihistamine	HCV	Chimeric mouse model	Entry?

S.NO	COMPOUND	STATUS/INDICATION	VIRUS	EXPERIMENTAL MODEL	TARGET
	FDA-Approved Synthetic drug candidates with repurposing potentials				
14.	Manidipine	Approved/antihypertensive	JEV, ZIKV	Infected cells in vitro, mouse model	NS4B
			HCMV,	Infected cells in vitro	IE2
15.	Favipiravir	Approved/antiviral	EBOV	Phase 2 clinical trial	RNA polymerase
16.	GS-5734	Investigational/antiviral	MERS- and SARS-CoV	Nonhuman primates	RNA polymerase
17.	Imatinib	Approved/anticancer	MERS- and SARS-CoV	Infected cells in vitro	Viral fusion
18.	Chlorpromazine	Approved/antipsychotic	MERS- and SARS-CoV	Infected cells in vitro	Undetermined
19.	Chlarithromycin/Naproxen + Oseltamivir	Approved/antibacterial, anti-inflammatory (+antiviral	Influenza	Phase 2b/3 clinical trials	Undetermined
20.	Nitazoxanide	Approved/antiparasitic	Influenza	Influenza	Maturation of hemagglutinin
			Rotavirus	Rotavirus	Viral morphogenesis
			Norovirus	Norovirus	Undetermined
21.	Raltegravir	Approved/antiviral	Herpesvirus	Infected cells in vitro	Terminase
22.	Lopinavir/ ritonavir + interferon b-1b	Approved/antiviral	MERS-CoV	Nonhuman primates, phase 2/3 clinical trial	Protease
23.	Lopinavir/ritonavir		HPV	Proof-of-concept clinical trial	Overexpression RNAse L and?
24.	Zidovudine	Cancer	AIDS	T-cell culture	Undetermined
25.	Minoxidi	Hypertension	Hair loss	Animal study	Undetermined
26.	Sildenafil	Angina	Erectile dysfunction	Animal study	Undetermined
27.	Thalidomid	Morning sickness	Erythema nodosum leprosum and multiple myeloma	Infected cells in vitro	Undetermined

DOI: http://dx.doi.org/10.5772/intechopen.102825

S.NO	COMPOUND	STATUS/INDICATION	VIRUS	EXPERIMENTAL MODEL	TARGET
	FDA-Approved Synthetic drug candidates with repurposing potentials				
44.	Danoprevir + ritonavir + interferon inhalation or lopinavir + ritonavir or TCM plus interferon inhalation	Protease inhibitors with cytokine as aerosol	COVID-19	Infected cells in vitro	Undetermined
45.	Xiyanping or lopinavir-ritonavirinterferon inhalation	Anti-inflammatory (Xiyanping) or Protease inhibitors with cytokine	COVID-19	Infected cells in vitro	Undetermined
46.	Xiyanping combined with lopinavir + ritonavir	Anti-inflammatory (Xiyanping) in combination with Protease inhibitors	COVID-19	Infected cells in vitro	Undetermined
47.	Combinations of oseltamivir, favipiravir, and chloroquine	Neuraminidase (Oseltamivir) in combination with antimalarial/ amebicide	COVID-19	Infected cells in vitro	Undetermined
48.	Vitamin C	Vitamin (Ascorbic acis)	COVID-19	Infected cells in vitro	Undetermined

Table 3.
Approved and candidate drugs with Re purposing potential as antiviral agents.

nonendemic geographical areas such as the USA and Europe. EBOV causes lethal sign and symptoms such as acute hemorrhage, fever, and 90% high fatality rate, it needs high-level biocontainment (BSL-4) which hamper the development of drugs and vaccines to act against EBOV hence no specific therapeutic agents are available yet. In this context, DR prompted the EBOV infection in the last outbreak which shows promising results to lethal the EBOV infection.

Drugs:

- This includes viral RNA polymerase inhibitors Favipiravir (Influenza A virus Japanese approved drug).
- GS-5734 adenosine analogs, amodiaquine, chloremiphene, toremifene, bepridil.
- In combination, DR treatment shows antiviral activity against EBOV but not approved regimen
- Targeted drug-combination approach results in the identification of toremifene–mefloquine–posaconazole and toremifene–clarithromycin–posaconazole, all previously identified by DR) that act synergistically in an EBOV (**Table 3**) entry-inhibition assay and at concentrations achievable in humans [5].

4. Drug repurposing in coronavirus

CoVs are RNA-viruses responsible for GIT respiratory and neurological disease in animals and zoonotic infection in humans, it has the potential to cross-species to species transmission in the domesticated animal which will become the source of spread in human. The major concern of outbreak is the morbidity and mortality of infection in human, and animal adaptability according to the physiological system and ability to upgrade itself to suppress the immune system which make life decline.

SARS-CoV is highly pathogenic it emerged in China in 2002/2003 with 8098 infections and 10% mortality, on the other hand in 2012 MERS-CoV outbreak spread to 27 countries so far by 35% mortality rate, to manage the threat of both the outbreaks by adopting three independent studies reporting an approach by DR for anti-CoV drug discovery were published, this methodology tested against MERS- and SARS-CoV, came up with the screening of dopamine receptor antagonist and antimalarials [6].

Drugs:

- FDA-approved drugs were tested against MERS- and SARS-CoV are dopamine receptor antagonist chlorpromazine and antimalarials chloroquine by DR-approach.
- The DR approach worked on ABL tyrosine kinase oncogene pathway which is essential for the entry of CoVS, whereas imatinib inhibits the replication of both MERS-and SARS-CoV, other host-targeting anti-CoV are Cyclophylin A, cyclosporin A, alispovir and cyclophilin A need further investigation.
- Other drug is in combination currently under clinical evaluation against MERS-CoV syndromes and now vaccines are available to control the SARS-CoV.

4.1 Drug repurposing in influenza and dengue

Influenza is an air-borne disease, belong to the family Orthomyxoviride and it causes a major pandemic outbreak. DR camping identified FDA-approved drugs which are under clinical evaluation with anti-influenza activity [7].

Drugs:

- The kinase inhibitors namely Dinaciclib, Flavopiridol, and PIK-75 reported to be highly effective H7N9, pdm H1N1, and H3N2.
- DR-approached inhibitors are Dapivirine, Naproxen, and antibiotic Clarithromycin.
- The three-drug combination therapy for the treatment of influenzas by targeting mutant viral neuraminidase Clarithromycin+ naproxen along with Oseltamivir was found to be very effective.
- Currently available repurposed drug for influenza treatment is anti-parasitic are nitazoxanide.

whereas Dengue virus (DENV) is a mosquito-borne disease, currently it is rapidly spreading important arthropod-born viral disease in the world. It requires the new drug to target the host cells, whereas the repurposing approach was found to be effective for therapeutic intervention.

Drugs:

- The viral protective inhibitors are Nelfinavir, Lopinavir, and Ritonavir are repurposed by *in silico* Drug design for DENV.
- Chloroquine has also proven the inhibition of type-2 replication in vero cells at a dose of 5 μg/ml by plaque assay qRT-PCR.
- Naturally effective alkaloids for the treatments are Castanospermine, cytomegalovirus against HIV-I, DENV-1, and in-vivo against herpes simplex & Raucher Murine Leukemia virus.
- Some chemotherapeutic agents like Dasatinib, Bortezomib, Prochlorperazin (Antipsychotic), Ivermectin, Suramin, Nitrazoxanide A (anti-parasitic) dexamethasone, Prednisolone (Steroids), Genteticin, Narasin and Minocycline (Antibiotic) [8].

5. Drug repurposing in DNA viruses (HIV, CMV, HSV, and HCV)

According to WHO, 26 million people have died due to HIV/AIDS in year 1981, and from 2018 till more than 1.10 million people were affected, this was the worst outbreak managed by hydroxy-chloroquine [9]. HCMV was the best example of host adaptation and the ability of virous to subvert, completely, cellular physiological processes in infected cells (**Table 3**).

Drugs:

- Anti-HCMV drugs are statin, cardiac glycosides & emetine (Anti-parasite).
- Kinase inhibitors Manidipine (anti-hypertensive) this drug modifies the host protein function and takes away from the viruses [10].
- Topical drugs such as Ciclopirox, olamine reduce replication of HSV-1 and HCV replication can be inhibited by Suberoylanilide, erlotinib, Dasatinib, and hydroxamic acid (anticancer drugs).
- Miscellaneous repurposed drugs are Ezetimibe (Cholesterol drug), Ferroquine (anti-malarial), Cyclizine, and phenothiazine (H1-antihistamine) [11].

6. Concluding remarks and future perspectives

Viral infectious diseases remain a major challenge due to the lack of specific medical regimen, to counteract the viral replication and pathogenesis required knowledge to understand the virus-host interaction and mutagenesis, which is now a days remain a puzzle for several known viral pathogens emerging as time and eternity. The development of a drug molecule which is able to target the exact replication is still remain challenging, to encounter the emerging new viral pathogenesis, in this context, DR or positioning approach on FDA-approved drug evaluation, reduce the risk for pipeline new drug discovery, with economic advantages and remarkable generation up to $25 billion annual sales.

The potentiality of the DR approach will target the host function as time and cost-effective route to develop the broad-spectrum antiviral, which already gave a positive outcome successfully by opening-up new pathways for viral infection. The drug repurposing approach feasibly worked on anticancer, antiviral, and antibacterial FDA-approved medicines, to counteract EBOV, MERS-CoV, SARS-CoV, COVID-19, and now a day to control newly emerging OMICRON. Moreover, the successful repurposing is based upon the concentrating required for antiviral activity, which is often higher than approved regimens. Reconsideration on regimen the combined dosage form will be more effective and feasible to reach the new target mentioned in (**Table 3**) [11]. The synergistic therapy will be the milestone formulation to combat EBOVA influenza and could also be the regimen to target other viral infections [12].

On the other hand, the combined formulation will be less toxic and the dose of the drug can also be minimized as compared to the approved formulation with less chances of drug resistance due to synergistic effect, [7, 13].

There is still to be vigilant: synergistic effect at low dose, medication required to interfere with each other to have different mechanism of action. The viral replication pathway or host needs to be targeted early, to inhibit the mutation with antiviral combination, finding the new approach might be the only possible way to encounter such kind of viral outbreak with different therapeutic intervention, it remains mandatory and can be addressed by DR (Drug Repurposing) or reprofiling camping. To overcome the drug discovery bottleneck for emerging and re-emerging viral infectious disease, even the more concerned one is death associated with COVID-19 and HIV, DR will be the major interest due to reduced failure rate and decreased time as well as resource consumptions, to be put forward the first HIV medicine innovated by DR which was initially used to treat cancer patient, this will be the millstone to turn the entire scenario tempted the researcher, during the global pandemic outbreak to design novel molecules by the re-tasking look on FDA-approved drugs.

Before reprofiling, it requires to be vigilant towards the challenges associated with the copyrights. This chapter represents the importance of research that need to be conducted by closing the leftover loops on FDA-approved drugs. The author was overwhelmed to represent the glimpse associated with reprofiling by putting it down, and look forward to work practically at YPCRC for fruitful future.

Acknowledgements

The author gratefully acknowledges the principle and management of Yenepoya Pharmacy College & Research Centre, Yenepoya University, Mangaluru, to carry out the work in the area of drug repurposing we look forward to do research on antiviral and antidiabetic domine.

Conflict of interest

The authors declare no conflict of interest.

Acronyms and abbreviations

DR	Drug Repurposing
CMV	Cytomegalovirus
HCMV	Human Cytomegalovirus
HCV	Hepatitis C Virus
EVD	Ebola Virous Disease
qRT-PCR	Quantitative Real-Time Polymerase Chain Reaction
RVFV	Rift Valley fever virus
MERS-CoV	Middle East Respiratory Syndrome Coronavirus
SARS-CoV	Severe Acute Respiratory Syndrome Coronavirus
EBOV	Ebola Virus
FDA	Food and Drug Administration
HIV	Human immunodeficiency Virus
AIDS	Acquired Immune Deficiency Syndrome
HSV	Herpes simplex Virus
DENV	Dengue Virus
H1N1, H3N2 & H7N9	Swine Flu Influenza
WHO	World Health Organization
M^{pro}	Main protease
Gly-fl-Ser/Gly/	Ala as motif cleavage
ABL tyrosine	Abelson murine Leukemia Viral gene

Reference tables

- Precedence and pitfalls of reprofiling candidates [13]
- Represents available library of vendors to be referred while designing and figuring out the Reprofiled candidate [14]
- Literature of successful repurposed candidates [15, 16].

Author details

Nikhat Farhana*, Mohammed Gulzar Ahmed, Mohammed Asif Iqbal, Nishmitha Gretta D'Souza, Sudhina Makuttan, Natasha Naval Aggarwal and Abdul Rahamanulla
Yenepoya Pharmacy College and Research Center, Department of Pharmaceutical Chemistry, Yenepoya (Deemed to be University), Derlakatte, Mangaluru, Karnataka, India

*Address all correspondence to: nik.nida13ada25@gmail.com

References

[1] Mani D, Wadhwani A, Krishnamurthy PT. Drug repurposing in antiviral research : A current scenario. Journal of Young Pharmacists. 2019;**11**(2):117-121

[2] Pizzorno A, Padey B, Terrier O, Rosa-calatrava M. Drug repurposing approaches for the treatment of influenza viral infection : Reviving old drugs to fight against a long-lived enemy. Journal of Young Pharmacists. 2019;**11**(2):117-121

[3] Mercorelli B, Palù G, Loregian A. Drug repurposing for viral infectious diseases : How far are we ? Trends in Microbiology. 2018;**26**(10):865-876. DOI: 10.1016/j.tim.2018.04.004

[4] Altay O, Mohammadi E, Lam S, Turkez H, Boren J, Nielsen J, et al. iScience ll current Status of COVID-19 therapies and drug repositioning applications. ISCIENCE. 2020;**23**(7): 101303. DOI: 10.1016/j.isci.2020.101303

[5] Sarkar A, Mandal K. Repurposing an antiviral drug against SARS-CoV-2 Main protease. Angew Chem Int Ed Engl. 2021 Oct 25;**60**(44):23492-23494

[6] Pushpakom S, Iorio F, Eyers PA, Escott KJ, Hopper S, Wells A, et al. Drug repurposing: Progress, challenges and recommendations. Nature Reviews Drug Discovery. 2018;**7**:234-238. DOI: 10.1038/nrd.2018.168

[7] Sultana J, Crisafulli S, Gabbay F, Lynn E, Shakir S. Challenges for drug repurposing in the COVID-19 pandemic era. Front. Pharmacol. 2020;**11**(November):1-13

[8] Yang C, Peng T, Hsu H, Lee Y, Wu S, Lin W, et al. ScienceDirect repurposing old drugs as antiviral agents for coronaviruses. Biomedical J. 2020;**3**:3-9

[9] Parnham MJ, Erakovic V, Giamarellos-bourboulis EJ, Perletti G, Verleden GM, Vos R. Pharmacology & Therapeutics Azithromycin : Mechanisms of action and their relevance for clinical applications. Pharmacology & Therapeutics. 2014;**143**(2):225-245. DOI: 10.1016/j.pharmthera.2014.03.003

[10] Rajkumar RP. Lithium as a candidate treatment for COVID-19: Promises and pitfalls. Drug Dev Res. 2020 Nov;**81**(7):782-785

[11] Cusinato J, Cau Y, Calvani AM, Mori M, Cusinato J, Cau Y, et al. Expert opinion on therapeutic patents repurposing drugs for the management of. Expert Opinion on Therapeutic Patents. 2021;**31**(4):295-308. DOI: 10.1080/13543776.2021.1861248

[12] Results ST. New England Journal. 2021;497-511

[13] Bauso LV, Imbesi C, Irene G, Cal G, Bitto A. New approaches and repurposed antiviral drugs for the treatment of the SARS-CoV-2 infection. Pharmaceuticals. 2021;**14**:1-19

[14] Swathi K, Nikitha B, Chandrakala B, Lakshmanadevi K, Malleswari M. Since January 2020 Elsevier has created a COVID-19 resource centre with free information in English and Mandarin on the novel coronavirus COVID- 19. The COVID-19 resource centre is hosted on Elsevier Connect, the company ' s public news and information. 2020;(January)

[15] Trivedi J, Mohan M. Drug repurposing approaches to combating viral infections. J Clin Med. 2020 Nov 23;**9**(11):3777

[16] Moleculer structure which have Repurpusing potential. Molecules. 2021;**24**(1):29-31